Update in Respiratory Diseases

Edited by Jose Carlos Herrera Garcia

Published in London, United Kingdom

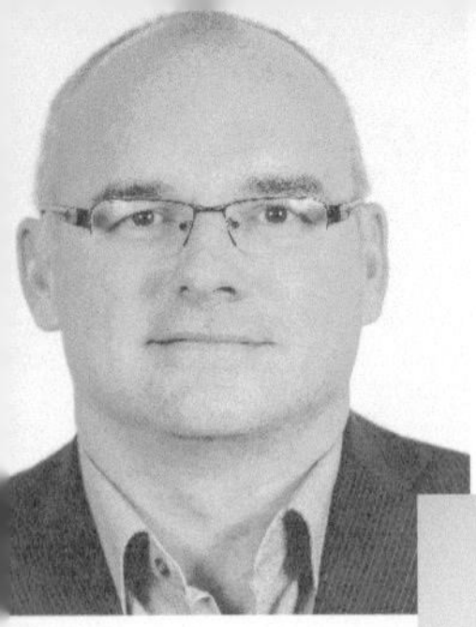
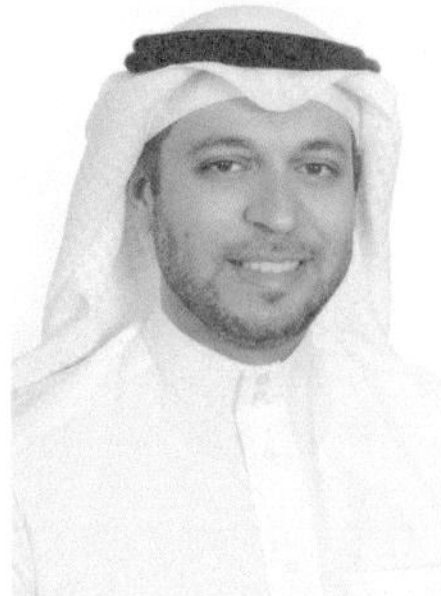
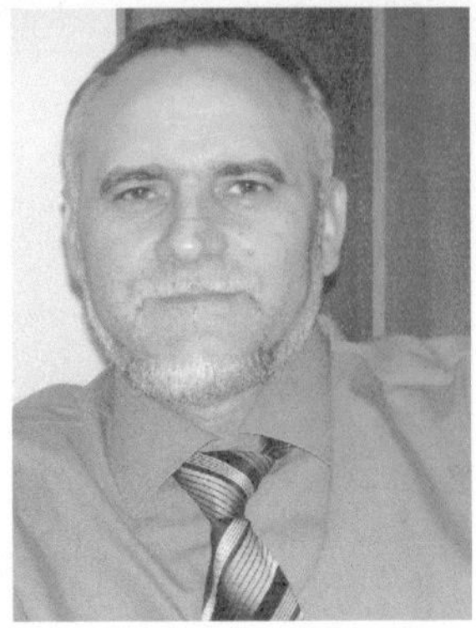
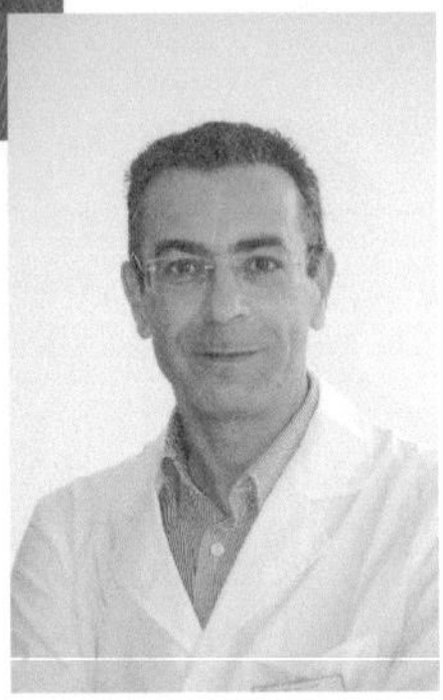
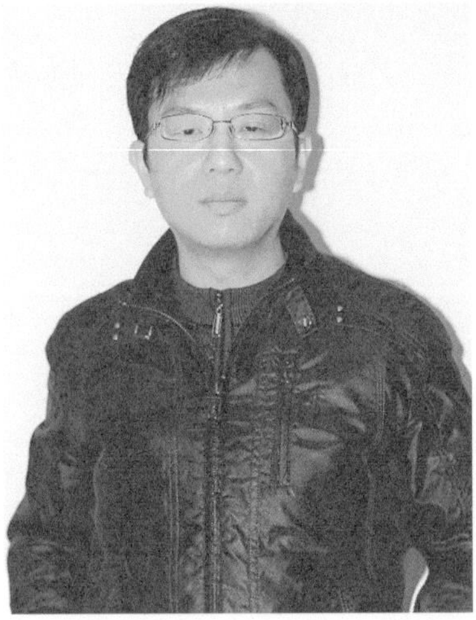
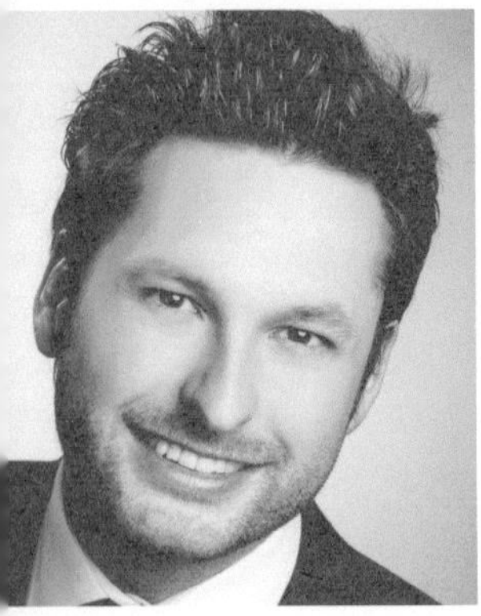
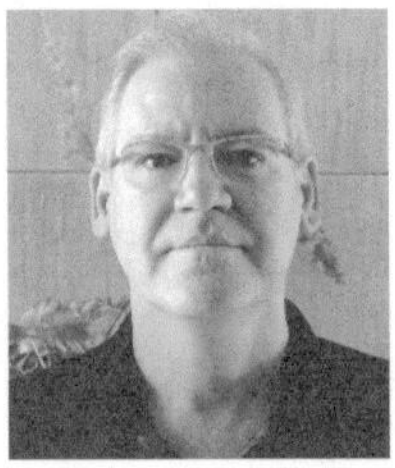

IntechOpen

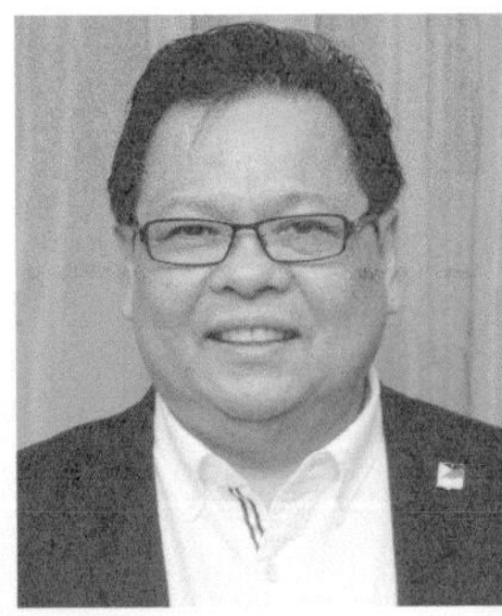
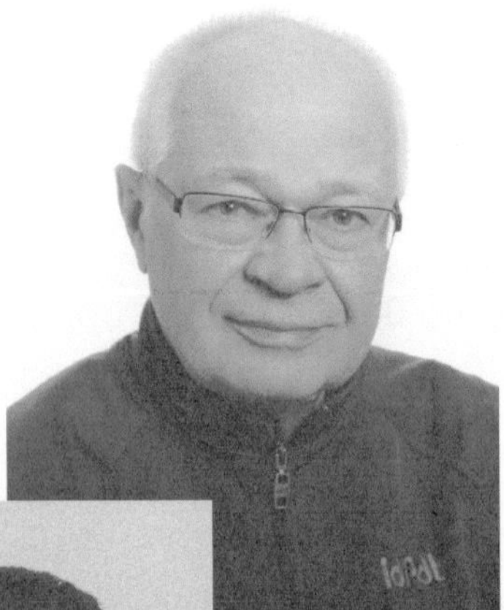
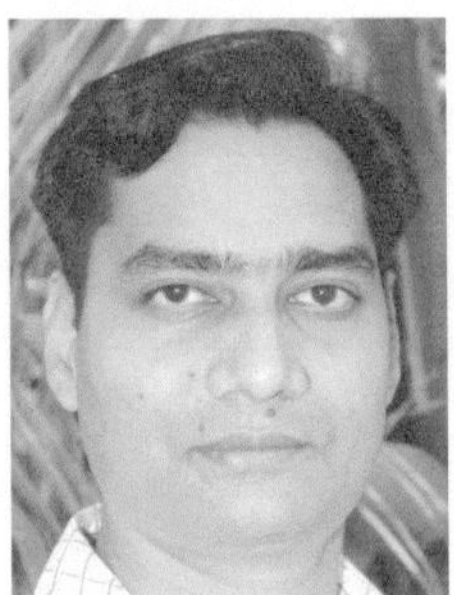
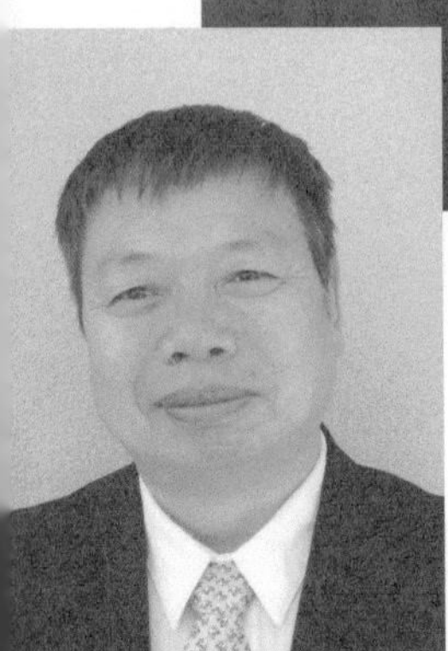
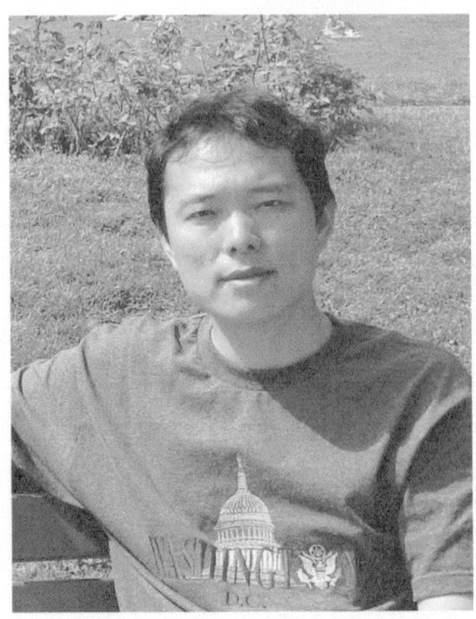
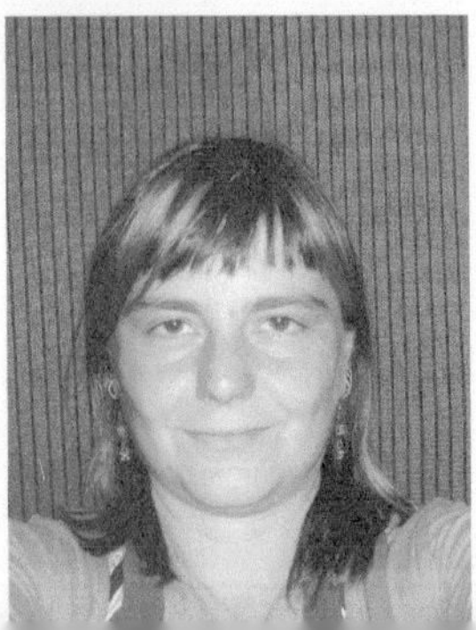

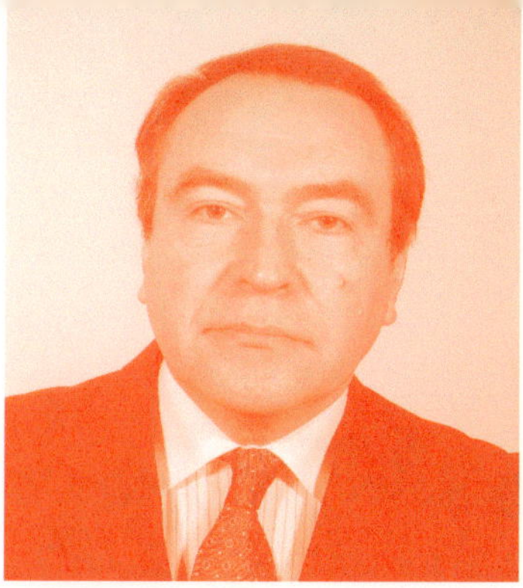
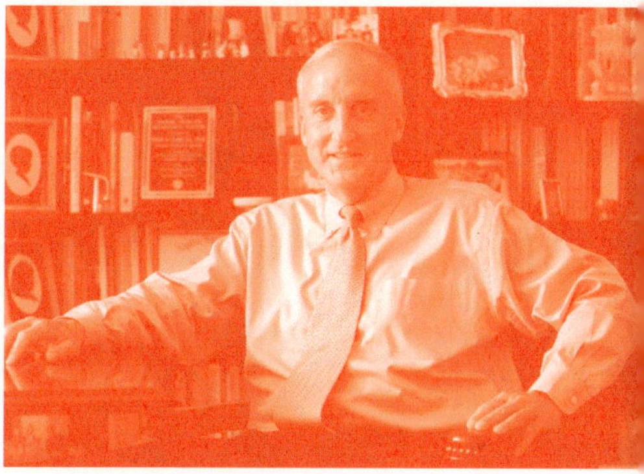
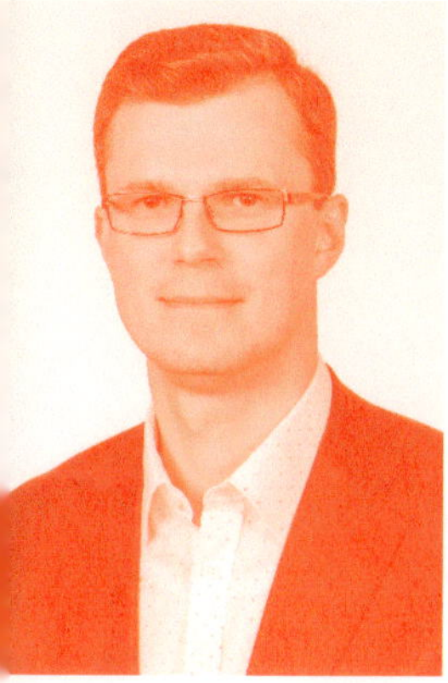
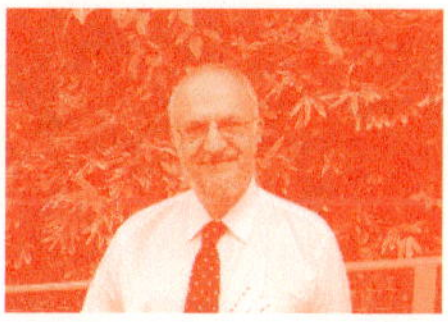
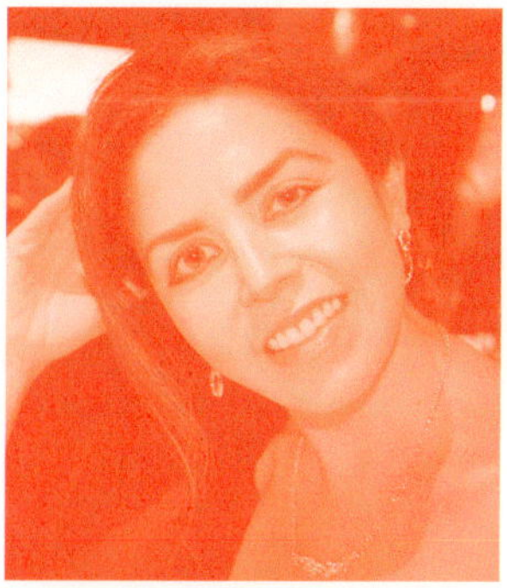

Supporting open minds since 2005

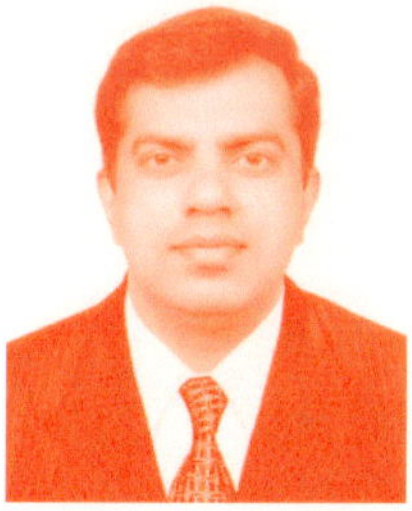
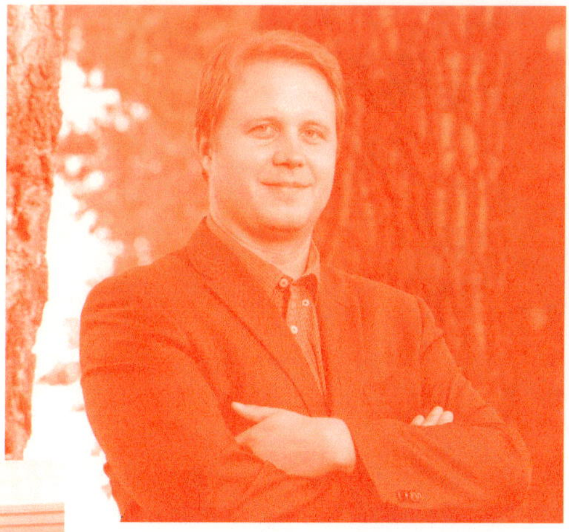
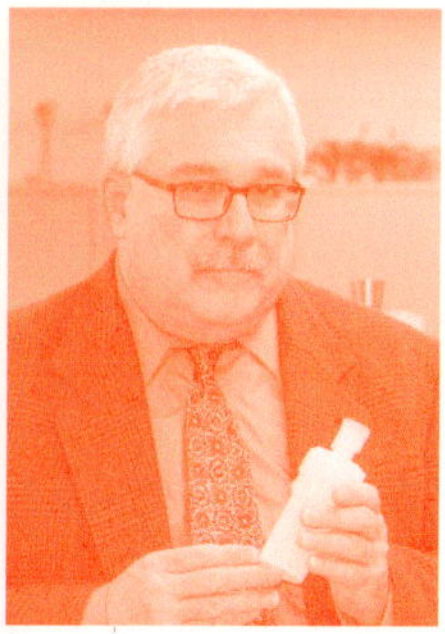
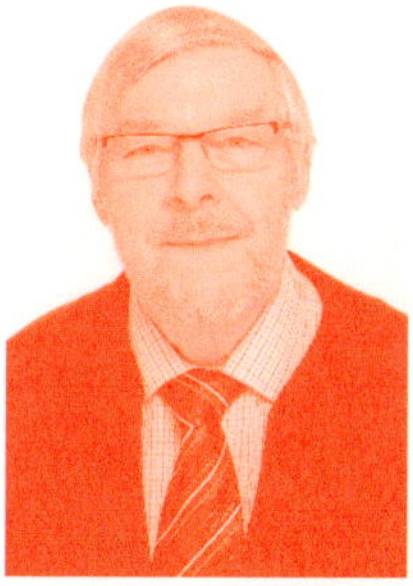
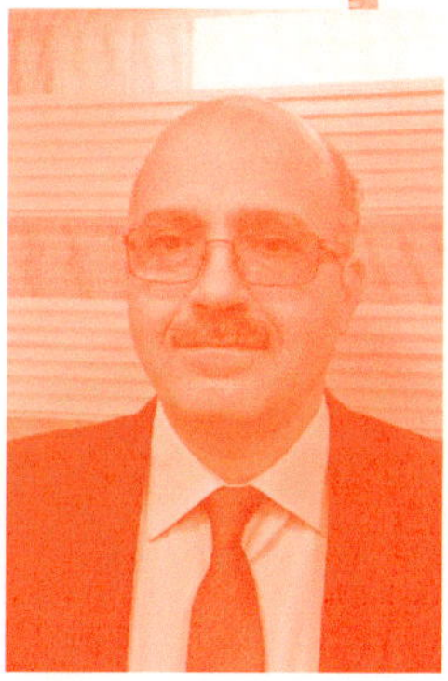
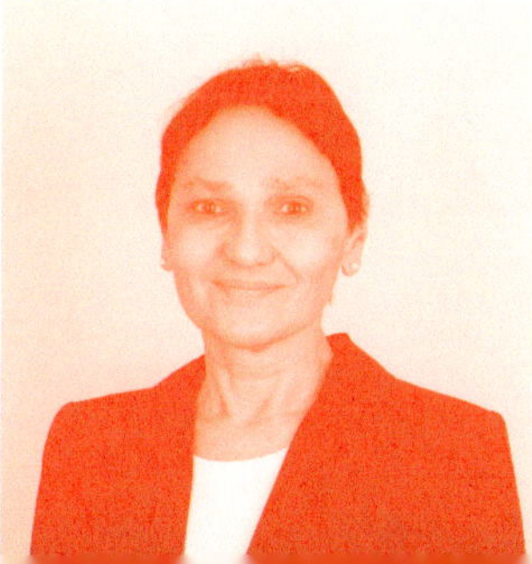
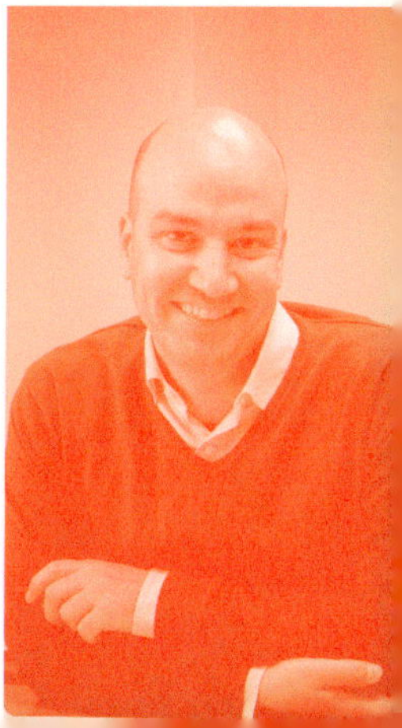

Update in Respiratory Diseases
http://dx.doi.org/10.5772/intechopen.77820
Edited by Jose Carlos Herrera Garcia

Contributors
Tomislav Jelic, Vera Nevzorova, Eugeny Gilifanov, Tatyana Brodskaya, Onix Cantres-Fonseca, Stefan-Marian Frent, Hulya Sahin, Jose Carlos Herrera Garcia, Nils-Tomas Delagar McBride, Rachit Shah, Alexander Maat, Ad Bogers, Amir Hossein Sadeghi, Edris Mahtab, Ting Zhou, You Shang, Yasser Ali Ali Kamal

First published in London, United Kingdom, 2020 by IntechOpen
IntechOpen is the global imprint of INTECHOPEN LIMITED, registered in England and Wales, registration number: 11086078, 5 Princes Gate Court, London, SW7 2QJ, United Kingdom
Printed in Croatia

British Library Cataloguing-in-Publication Data
A catalogue record for this book is available from the British Library

Additional hard and PDF copies can be obtained from orders@intechopen.com

Update in Respiratory Diseases
Edited by Jose Carlos Herrera Garcia
p. cm.
Print ISBN 978-1-83880-894-5
Online ISBN 978-1-83880-895-2
eBook (PDF) ISBN 978-1-83880-896-9

For EU product safety concerns:
IN TECH d.o.o., Prolaz Marije Krucifikse Kozulić 3, 51000 Rijeka, Croatia, info@intechopen.com or visit our website at intechopen.com.

Meet the editor

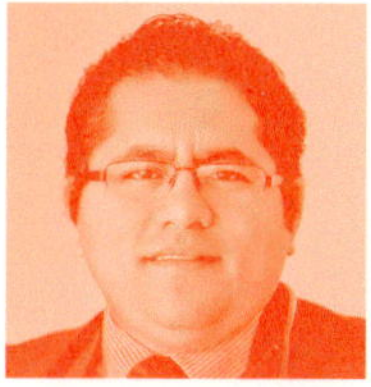

José Carlos Herrera García is a physician specialist in pneumology and internal medicine with a Master's in health administration. He is a research author of multiple national and international articles and a speaker in the field. He has authored book notes on pulmonology for undergraduate studies and many chapters on the specialist field of pulmonology. He is a doctor dedicated to the clinic, teaching, and research. He currently works as a medical specialist in the city of Puebla, Mexico. He is certified by the Council of Pulmonology and Thorax Surgery and is a Member of the Latin American Association of Thorax (ALAT) and the European Respiratory Society (ERS). He is the author of several national and international articles, focused on his specialty and has publications in the field of asthma, COPD and pulmonary hypertension. He is the Deputy Chief of Residents in the specialty of pulmonology and Chief of Residents in the specialty of internal medicine in Medica Sur Mexico City,

Contents

Preface

This book describes the latest developments in the field of pulmonology, in discussing what is new in the field of respiratory medicine, thoracic surgery, and advances in chronic diseases. The chapters are perfectly written for your understanding and especially for the updating of pneumologists who require a brief and concise update in these times. It is very gratifying for me to be the editor-in-chief of this edition that for the moment fills me with pride to be part of this text, together with other outstanding physicians in pulmonary medicine. I am infinitely grateful to all the collaborators for their effort and dedication to each chapter of the book that you will like for the ease of reading in these bulging times of medicine. I can only say that I appreciate all the support that was given to me in this excellent update on respiratory medicine, commanded by a Mexican doctor.

Jose Carlos Herrera Garcia
Unidad de Funcion Pulmonar SC,
Puebla, México

Section 1

Asthma and COPD

Chapter 1

Eosinophils as a Biomarker in Asthma and COPD

Jose Carlos Herrera Garcia

Abstract

Asthma and COPD are two diseases related to eosinophils. But at present, we do not know with certainty how much these cells participate in these diseases, beyond that the treatment of the underlying cause produces the resolution of eosinophilia in a "reactive" way. Eosinophil-related diseases are a spectrum of systemic diseases such as Asthma and COPD in pneumology area. Under inflammatory conditions, the number of circulating eosinophils or tissues can increase dramatically, with rapid development of eosinophilia and we can obtain in a simple laboratory test. In general, the number of eosinophils in the blood can provide useful information and considering the differential diagnosis and for the subsequent test of patients presenting with eosinophilia. The treatment of eosinophilia currently in number of 300 cells in which is the criteria and the target to be treat. The best known and most used of all treatments for diseases related to eosinophils are corticosteroids, which decrease circulating and tissue eosinophils in a few hours, through mechanisms that include the direct activation of eosinophil program death. Targeted treatment against eosinophils could improve airway remodeling through mechanisms that are not fully known, and their effects on lung function are variable and decreasing symptoms in patients.

Keywords: eosinophil, asthma, COPD

1. Introduction

Asthma and COPD are two diseases related to eosinophils in which eosinophils are the main cause and journals have evidence an increase in their number in the blood with or without evidence of their activation. But at present, we do not know with certainty how much these cells participate in these diseases, beyond that the treatment of the underlying cause produces the resolution of eosinophilia in a "reactive" way. Eosinophil-related diseases are a spectrum of systemic diseases such as Asthma and COPD in pneumology area. Even within the principal diseases related to eosinophils, the location, type of tissue involved, and magnitude of eosinophilia vary greatly. Under inflammatory conditions, the number of circulating eosinophils or tissues can increase dramatically, with rapid development of eosinophilia and we can obtain in a simple laboratory test. In general, the number of eosinophils in the blood can provide useful information and considering the differential diagnosis and for the subsequent test of patients presenting with eosinophilia. Currently eosinophils has taken a very important role in the treatment of severe diseases, we know are so prevalent and increased morbidity and mortality in serious phases which produce a lower quality of life in patients, the treatment of eosinophilia currently in number of 300 cells in which is the criteria and the target to be treat. The best known and most used of all treatments for diseases related to eosinophils are corticosteroids, which decrease circulating and tissue eosinophils in a few hours, through mechanisms that include the direct activation of eosinophil program death. But, under certain circumstances, eosinophils can become resistant to these drugs or in the presence of high levels of eosinophil survival cytokines, such as IL-5 by example. With the administration of anti-IL-5 antibodies, such as mepolizumab or reslizumab the blood eosinophils typically decrease by at least 80% within a few days, without decreasing them much in the tissues, such as in the lower airways. Asthma, presumably due to the action of other eosinophil cytokines, such as GM-CSF, present in tissues. Comparatively, the administration of benralizumab, an anti-IL-5 antibody that acts on the IL-5 receptor, causes a much deeper and longer decrease in eosinophils, by activating antibody-dependent cellular cytotoxicity. Targeted treatment against eosinophils in eosinophilic asthma and eosinophilic COPD decreases exacerbations and could improve airway remodeling through mechanisms that are not fully known, and their effects on lung function are variable and decreasing symptoms in patients.

Data from multiple studies in asthma and eosinophilic COPD suggest that they are safe long-term drugs despite the decrease in eosinophils over time, as well as being well tolerated. Eosinophils exist in virtually all vertebrates as part of the innate immune system, which underscores the important benefits they must provide to their guests. In humans, they are in normal ranges when their blood levels are <500 / μL, although this number can vary between 350 to 600 depending on the laboratory. Eosinophilia is defined when its number is>300/μL in the recent studies and guidelines [1, 2].

2. Eosinophil hematopoiesis

For eosinophils to develop, a unique set of transcription factors is required, which if not present, do not develop (**Figure 1**). Similarly, the eosinophil lineage

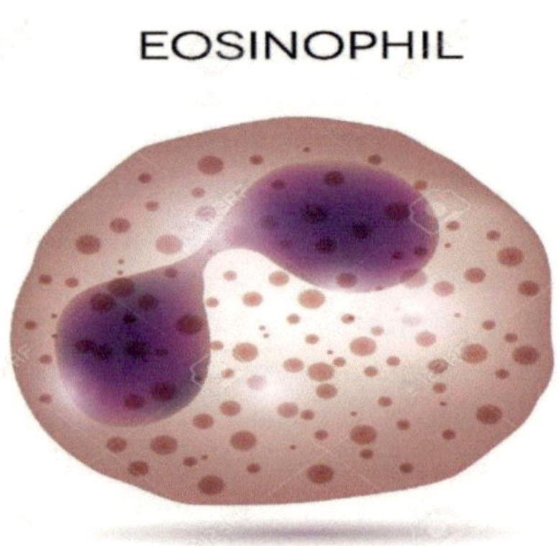

Figure 1.
The eosinophil.

depends on the appearance of a specific receptor on its surface for IL-5. The expression on the cell surface of the IL-5 receptor is one of the first events for the development of the specific eosinophil lineage that occurs in the bone marrow, although recent data in rats suggest that another cytokine, the IL- 13, has a role in increasing the differentiation of eosinophils at a point "upstream" to that of IL-5. Although the source of IL-5 and IL-33 within the bone marrow necessary for the development of eosinophils is not known exactly, it is likely that T cells and certain innate lymphoid cells (CLI2) are the important sources, at least for IL-5 [2].

3. Beneficial functions of eosinophils in homeostasis and host defense

Most of what is known about eosinophils in terms of their roles in health and homeostasis, comes from data obtained from animal studies. It is believed that eosinophils contribute a large amount of beneficial substances that help in the development, remodeling, and tissue repair. Their roles in innate and adaptive immune responses include the favorable influence on the development of immune cells, provide antibacterial, antifungal, and antiviral responses and help control glucose metabolism, myocyte regeneration, lean fat development and adiposity. Most of these functions have been demonstrated in animal models, so their reality in humans is uncertain. In addition, although the very important role of eosinophils during type 2 immune responses against helminths and other parasitic infections is considered almost dogmatic, their total certainty in humans is controversial because in many patients in pandemic parasitic infections we know have increase eosinophils and we do not the normal range in laboratory test and the main changes that decreasing of increasing (**Figure 2**). Therefore, despite the growing interest in knowing what eosinophils actually in the immune system and in disease circumstance, in the nest days we need to know and much remains to be investigated [3].

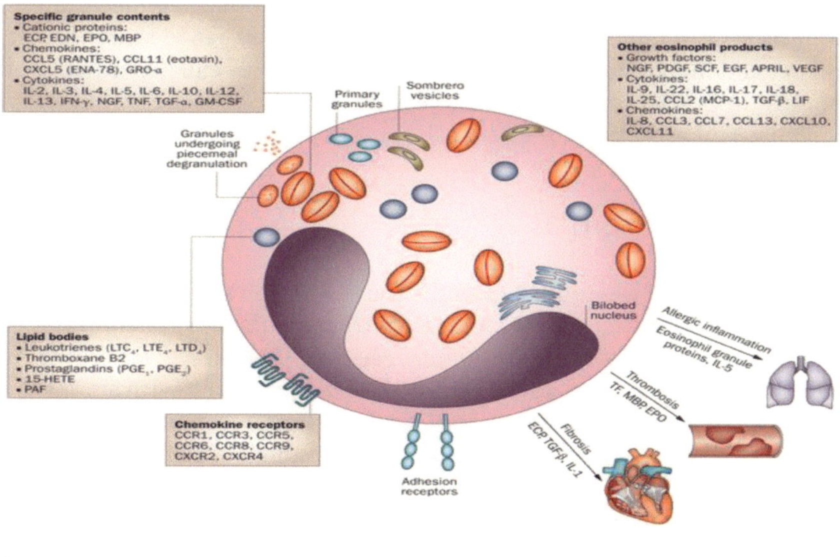

Figure 2.
The eosinophil cycle and function.

4. Asthma and COPD

COPD and asthma have a pathogenic and pathophysiological basis easily differentiable in most cases. They also share a series of clinical similarities that often make their differentiation complex, especially in-patient smokers with a history of atopy and eosinophilia. But we have patients with combined symptoms and different phenotypic. The characteristics clinics shared by both diseases are based on inflammation and airway obstruction, now we know in certain papers that COPD is a fibrotic disease but when the patient have some allergic characteristics the disease is like an inflammatory problem and the eosinophils have a role in both. The incomplete reversible and progressive in COPD and variable and reversible in asthma. Also, the location of the inflammatory response in these pathologies also have differences, allowing to locate the predominant involvement of COPD in the peripheral airway and in the pulmonary parenchyma, in contrast to the respect of pulmonary parenchyma and panfocal airway involvement in asthma. The cell count obtained from bronchioalveolar lavage (BAL), induced sputum and bronchial biopsies in patients with COPD demonstrate the predominant presence of neutrophils, CD8 + T lymphocytes and abundant macrophages. In asthma, eosinophils, mast cells, CD4 + T cells and fewer macrophages meet in samples representative of the tracheobronchial tree, but there are some patients with paucigranulocitic phenotypic. Inflammatory mediators also differ, playing a predominant role leukotriene-B4 (LTB4), interleukin 8 (IL-8) and tumor necrosis factor alpha (TNF-α), among others, in the case of COPD, while in asthma have found multiple inflammatory variables, represented for histamine, leukotrienes and interleukins 4 and 5.

The fraction of exhaled nitric oxide in patients with asthma is found increased, reflecting the greater eosinophilic inflammation. Thus, it seems reasonable to define a high Th2 patient profile in a non-invasive way by using indirect markers such as IgE > 100 IU and blood eosinophils>300 cells/microliter, or eosinophils in sputum>3%. Along these lines, a recent study has shown that eosinophilia together with elevated levels of periostin was the best predictor of improvement in lung function in COPD patients treated for three months with inhaled corticosteroids and LABA. However, it seems that a more integrative approach, which unites clinical features and molecular mechanisms, is the best way to identify disease sub phenotypes and individualized treatments. The fraction of exhaled nitric oxide is poor studied in COPD, and we know there is not a confinable test to follow a patient we do not have inflammation or have both [3].

5. Eosinophils and COPD

In December 2017, we published in the journal Respirar de ALAT, a manuscript of the study findings of 50 Mexican patients in the outpatient pulmonology clinic at the University Hospital of Puebla, Mexico, the results were prevalence of eosinophilia (74% women and 26% men). 50% associated with smoking and 50% with exposure to biomass. 36% presented representative eosinophilia which indicated the relevance of this marker taking into account that 50% of all the patients studied were in GOLD IVD stage. Tine and colleagues pointed out that blood eosinophils may have a paradoxical benefit for COPD patients; In patients with blood eosinophil counts of 2% or more versus patients with counts of less than 2%, better lung function, better quality of life, fewer symptoms and less comorbidities have been reported. It has also been shown that the risk of pneumonia, regardless of the use of inhaled steroids, is lower in patients with eosinophil blood counts of 2% or more. These facts suggest, the authors wrote, that the use of eosinophil-targeted therapies can actually be detrimental to COPD patients [4, 5].

6. Eosinophilic pathways in asthma

The Eosinophils nowadays are the most inflammatory status seen in asthma, in patients that have persistent eosinophilic airway inflammation is a severe status in some cases. Because these patients have neutrophilic or paucigranulocytic count and separate in allergic and nonallergic patients with severe symptoms. The pathways for eosinophil recruitment are quite distinct. Allergic eosinophilic asthma is driven by Th2 lymphocytes. Allergens, presented to naive CD4+ T cells by dendritic cells, induce differentiation toward Th2 cells, which produce IL4, IL5 and leading to IgE class to airway eosinophilia and mucous hypersecretion. In nonallergic eosinophilic asthma, epithelium-derived cytokines (IL25, IL33, TSLP) are released in response to air pollutants, microbes or glycolipids (**Figure 3**). These bind to receptors on type-2 innate lymphoid cells (ILC2s), activating them to produce the Th2-associated cytokines IL5 and IL13, which lead to eosinophilia, mucous hypersecretion and airway hyper-reactivity, in the majority of allergic asthma cases, the presence of eosinophils may be a secondary consequence of the allergic cascade that recruits them to the site of inflammation in the evolution of the disease. In some patients, however, particularly those with severe, non-allergic asthma the eosinophil may play a more central role, possibly initiating the disease or persistent disease or persistent symptoms, these patients are typically older women with comorbid nasal polyps, aspirin sensitivity and late-onset asthma concluded in a different phenotypic [5].

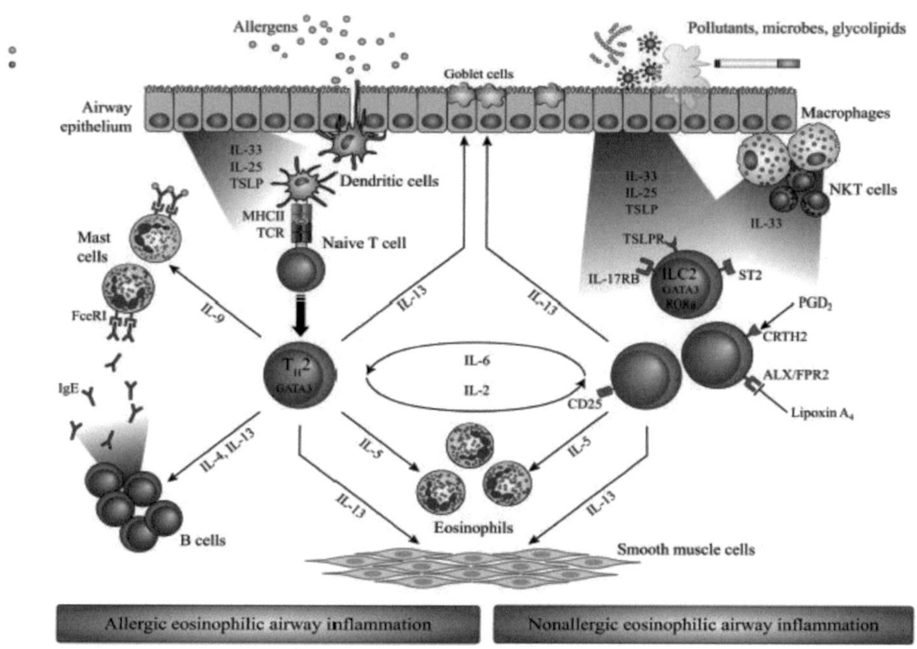

Figure 3.
Allergic and non-allergic eosinophilic pathways in asthma.

7. Eosinophilic inflammation in COPD

In COPD, inflammation is more commonly associated with T helper 1 lymphocyte (Th1)-mediated immunity driven by neutrophils, often in response to bacterial colonization. However, as with asthma, COPD presents as a number of different clinical phenotypes and, in around 10–40% of patients, a degree of eosinophilic inflammation is present during stable state. We published some cases with severe COPD versus health patients in a asthma clinic in Puebla, and we describe that we do not know when is the time to take a eosinophils sample and make a different diagnosis in the clinic, the patients came to take a sample in stable state and have minor eosinophils cells like health people, and concluded like we need to know when is the better time to take a eosinophils sample. The cell senescence likely plays a pathophysiological role in COPD (**Figure 4**) particularly in relation to the release of cytokines other factors from senescent cells, many of which are also implicated in the pathogenesis of COPD [5].

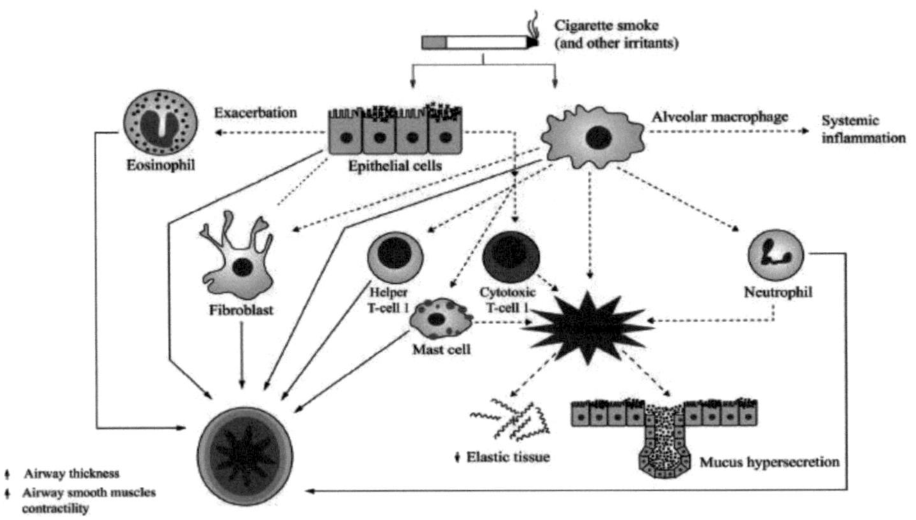

Figure 4.
Relationship between airway inflammation and bronchial abnormalities in COPD.

8. The utility of measuring blood eosinophil levels in asthma and COPD

The most important point in this chapter is the utility of measuring blood eosinophils as a biomarker to treatment in stable or exacerbating COPD. Blood eosinophil levels can either be expressed as an absolute count (150 cells) or as a percentage, actually there are many groups that define them, like <2%, ≥2–<3%, ≥3–<4%, <150 cells·μL − 1, 150–<300 cells·μL − 1, ≥300–<400 cells and ≥ 400 cells were used in the post hoc analysis of WISDOM. 2020 guidelines from the Global Initiative for Chronic Obstructive Lung Disease (GOLD) have recommended blood eosinophil counts ≥300 cells in stable COPD as the diagnostic criterion for initiating therapy with ICS/long-acting β-agonist (LABA). However, eosinophilia is defined, the utility of the measurement is limited by the stability of the measurement. People with COPD often start treatment with Dual Therapy (LABA/LAMA) some people use monotherapy in some patients, but in some group of patients continue use inhaled corticosteroids like added, sure measuring the number of eosinophils and concluded the people who will benefit with this kind of therapy. Some patients experience a worsening of their symptoms known as an exacerbation and the eosinophils maybe predict the risk of exacerbations that is so important for clinicians treating this patients, but there is a pooled analysis in 2020 with Singh et al. concluded that in a pooled analysis of 22,125 patients with COPD, do not find a clinically important relationship between baseline blood eosinophils count and exacerbation rate and is not a clinically useful predictor of future exacerbation risk, I think maybe we can use in worsening symptoms in a single time of the life of the patient, COPD is dynamic and heterogenic disease, maybe we can use in some cases in which the patient worsening symptoms [6].

The utility of measuring blood eosinophils to guide therapy is likely to vary depending upon the clinical status of the patient, i.e. whether their COPD is stable, or they are experiencing an exacerbation. Now in press we have a manuscript that we can show in a cohort with severe COPD patients and healthy controls the blood eosinophils count do not change in a single sample and the count was similar in the same group in the same time. The evidence suggests that measuring, eosinophil levels to help guide therapy is useful with measuring eosinophils count to use ICS/ LABA, and reduction the use of inhaled corticosteroids y some patients that do not need this treatment. In COPD we need to consider the eosinophil count to choose treatment [6].

9. We can use eosinophils like a target and biomarker in the biologics era

Anti-IL5 therapies are a great promise in patients with eosinophilic asthma, and we do not know if is the same to COPD, suggesting that depletion of eosinophils may not be a valid target in COPD. An initial study using the anti-IL5R antibody, benralizumab, in COPD patients with elevated baseline sputum eosinophils ($\geq$3%) demonstrated numerical improvements in exacerbation rates, SGRQ-C and the self-administered Chronic Respiratory Questionnaire (CRQ-SAS) scores, and FEV1 (fraction exhalation volume in 1 second) however, these improvements were not statistically significant. Mepolizumab significantly reduced sputum and blood eosinophil counts compared with placebo in COPD patients with raised baseline eosinophils but, again, these differences did not translate into significant between-group differences in lung function parameters, exacerbation rates, and health-related quality of life. The role of eosinophils in COPD is complex and the benefits observed with ICS (inhaled Corticosteroids) are likely related to their effects on cells or pathways that do not involve eosinophils. These results suggest a potential role for eosinophilic airway inflammation on COPD exacerbations, but also clearly underline the fact that further studies are needed to refine the patients who may benefit from eosinophil-targeted treatments in COPD. The Benefit–risk ratio of ICS in patients with COPD based on blood eosinophil level in stable disease with increasing eosinophils counts, the use of ICS may offer increased benefit by reducing COPD exacerbations and always have precaution for development a pneumonia. ICS use in patients with lower eosinophils counts is potentially associated with decreased benefit and increased risk of pneumonia. Celli comment that the possibility that an easily obtained biomarker such as peripheral blood eosinophil count may help determine a patient's risk for certain outcomes and likelihood of responding to specific therapy is very appealing. However, as in many areas in life, "the devil is in the details", and more data is needed before blood eosinophil levels can be used to identify a COPD phenotype amenable to specific immunomodulatory therapy [7].

10. Variability of blood eosinophils as a biomarker in asthma and COPD

Peter G. Gibson et al. described to consider are those that lower the count and could lead to a false-negative test for diagnosis of the eosinophilic phenotype. These include eating, exercise, medications, and the time of testing. Consuming a light meal was found to reduce blood eosinophils between 2 and 4 h after eating, with an average 23% reduction at 4 h (from 130 to 100 cells/μL). Exercise also reduces blood eosinophil counts. For example, a symptom-limited exercise test in COPD patients reduced blood eosinophils at 2 h, with normalization by 24 h. In Puebla, Mexico in 2019 we compared two groups of patients in Asthma and COPD clinic, this two groups were: One group of severe COPD patients [6] and other group healthy subjects [6] workers for the clinic, the age of the patient were 45–60 years and we found that the eosinophil count was similar in the COPD group and the control group. A study was carried out in the Asthma and COPD clinic of the City of Puebla in a Private Angeles Hospital, the presence of two groups of patients with COPD and another as a control group of health workers, and we obtained very interesting data from the account of the eosinophils in a stable state of the patients, since they came voluntarily on a normal and stable day to take the eosinophil count and what were our results: the following: 2 groups of patients with COPD 1 group with 6 patients and the second group with 8 healthy workers. The patients with COPD were severe but in a stable and controlled state and presented an eosinophil count between 144 to 240 cells, and the group of health workers with an eosinophil range between 102 and 192 cells. This finding in this small cohort of patients as a pilot study allows us to see that patients with severe COPD may have low eosinophil ranges because they are stable and controlled just like healthy workers and subsequently be able to use the eosinophil range in some exacerbation of patients who may present an increase in eosinophils and change the therapy, this small work carried out in a particular clinic allows us to conclude that serious patients who have a stable state really have eosinophils in the normal range and the increase of 300 cells is really a figure in which We can make changes in therapy, but on the other hand, in stable patients, it would not be appropriate to take hematic biometry in the stability consultations because it would not be case knowing that the eosinophil count remains normal and only in an exacerbation take them to determine changes in current therapeutics. We concluded that in asthma patients the eosinophil count is variable than the COPD patients [8–10].

11. What is the utility of eosinophils in two prevalent respiratory diseases today?

As described earlier in this chapter, eosinophils are in these times of progress in the treatment of asthma and COPD one of the important pillars at different stages of the disease, as described earlier, approximately 4 years ago we did not have a marker that we allow you to change our decisions in the therapy of these patients in the stable phase or in exacerbations, it seems that its use is very bleak in stable patients, but already established a little more scientific in its use in exacerbations, every patient shows us one of the possible use of eosinophils in the whole path of the disease either in a stable phase or in exacerbation. In the definition of the disease its integration is clearly not useful, as well as in the epidemiological phase, but not in the diagnostic phase where it can be important to emphasize the phenotypes in the two diseases such as in asthma: eosinophilic asthma and in COPD as eosinophilic COPD. In the clinic it has not contributed great importance and we do not think it is relevant to know eosinophilia to determine if it is asthma or COPD even the spirometry is still the most important pillar of the diagnosis. in the classification of the disease it is of the utmost importance to determine if it is stable or exacerbated, as well as in the treatment that is vital to start steroid treatment, we know in asthma it is the pillar treatment of the disease not so in COPD but it allows to differentiate those responders to corticosteroids. Eosinophils at present and thanks to studies we can clearly establish its use at the beginning of the use of some biological medication to those patients with severe or exacerbated disease, as you know the exacerbations are those that deteriorate the disease and give a poor prognosis. As biomarker for biological initiation it is vital, as it has also been demonstrated in its use in the follow-up of patients, as part of the response to the treatment already established. There are still unknowns about the use of these cells in stable patients, we are developing a writing of the results of a pilot work on the values of eosinophils in stable patients with serious disease and healthy patients, these results will be shortly where we can show that in the stable patient there is still controversy in the use of treatment in patients with eosinophilia [10].

12. Conclusion

Asthma and COPD are two chronic diseases linked to exacerbations and possible quality of life of patients, the introduction of eosinophils as biomarkers in the evolution of the disease has opened a promising panorama as a biomarker in the classification of patients, their severity, prognosis and presence of exacerbations. Eosinophilia in these diseases is a reality and as pulmonologists we have a duty to always carry out that scrutiny that allows us to characterize our patients and to prescribe the appropriate treatment always taking into account the possible use of biologists in patients with severe disease. Both asthma and COPD are complex, heterogeneous conditions comprising a wide range of phenotypes, some of which are refractory to currently available treatments. These phenotypes and identification of biomarkers with which to recognize to guide an appropriate treatment for researchers and clinicians. The potential of blood eosinophils nowadays has potential and much attention in medical research to choose the optimal and correct treatment. In asthma, the rationale for their use as such is more clearly defined, with several well-controlled studies demonstrating that patients with higher eosinophil counts are prone to more severe disease and poorer outcomes. As a result, new biologic therapies have been developed to tailor treatment to these patients. In COPD, high blood eosinophil counts may predict a favorable response to ICS on top of LABA/LAMA, especially in patients with a history of frequent exacerbations, but the exact position and the definition of clinically significant eosinophilia is need to be more studied for the use of blood eosinophils for the identification of patients who may benefit from targeted treatments (**Table 1**). the use of eosinophils in clinical practice in COPD needs to be evaluated in prospective studies before firm conclusion and demonstrated in stable patients [10]. Eosinophilic inflammation is a stable longitudinal phenotype in a substantial proportion of COPD patients, which can be predicted over 12 months by an initial blood level measurement. The need for biomarkers to identify patients who may benefit from treatments in airways disease. As more treatment options are becoming available, we need to research and choose the biomarkers like elements or activation states of eosinophilic inflammation and will support the selection of treatment we need to control the patient in asthma and COPD. These events are seasonal in nature and relate to bacterial etiology and considerate the weather to take the sample [11].

Utility	Asthma	COPD
In definition	–	–
In epidemiological decision	–/+	–
In diagnosis	+/–	–
In clinic	+	+
In classification	+	–
In exacerbations	+	+
In treatment	++	++
In biological treatment	+++	+
Following	++	+
Stable	+	+/–

Table 1.
Utility of eosinophil as a biomarker in clinic.

Author details

Jose Carlos Herrera Garcia
Unidad de Funcion Pulmonar SC, Puebla, Mexico

*Address all correspondence to: jchg10@yahoo.com.mx

References

[1] Konstantinos Kostikas, Caterina Brindicci and Francesco Patalano: Blood Eosinophils as Biomarkers to Drive Treatment Choices in Asthma and COPD: *Current Drug Targets,* 2018, *19,* 1882-1896.

[2] Bruce S. Bochner: The Eosinophil: for better or worse, in sickness and in health: Ann Allergy Asthma Immunol. 2018 August; 121(2): 150-155. doi:10.1016/j.anai.2018.02.031.

[3] Peter G. Gibson: in Variability of blood eosinophils as a biomarker in asthma and COPD: Respirology (2018) 23, 12-13 doi: 10.1111/resp.13200.

[4] Herrera-García JC and cols: Prevalencia de eosinofilia y características clínicas en una cohorte de pacientes con EPOC en un Hospital de Tercer Nivel de Puebla: Respirar 2018 Volumen 10: número 1: Página 25

[5] Long Gabriella H and cols: Letter to editor: The stability of blood Eosinophils in chronic obstructive pulmonary disease: Respiratory Research (2020) 21:15 https://doi.org/10.1186/s12931-020-1279-4.

[6] Tine M, Biondini D, Semenzato U, et al. Reassessing the role of eosinophils as a biomarker in chronic obstructive pulmonary disease. J Clin Med. doi: 10.3390/jcm8070962.

[7] Dave Singh, Jadwiga A. Wedzicha, Salman Siddiqui, Alberto de la Hoz, Wenqiong Xue, Helgo Magnussen, Marc Miravitlles, James D. Chalmers and Peter M. A. Calverley. (2020). Blood eosinophils as a biomarker of future COPD exacerbation risk: pooled data from 11 clinical trials. (2020) 21:240, *Respiratory Research*. https://doi.org/10.1186/s12931-020-01482-1

[8] Oliver B, Tonga K, Darley D, et al. COPD treatment choices based on blood eosinophils: are we there yet? Breathe 2019;15: 318-323.

[9] Negewo et al: Peripheral blood eosinophils: a surrogate marker for airway eosinophilia in stable COPD: International Journal of COPD 2016:11 1495-1504.

[10] Bartolome Celli: Is the Blood Eosinophil Count a Useful Biomarker in COPD? The devil is in the Details!: *Arch Bronconeumol. 2017;*53(8)*:415-416.*

[11] Kim VL, Coombs NA, Staples KJ, et al. Impact and associations of eosinophilic inflammation in COPD: analysis of the AERIS cohort. Eur Respir J 2017; 50: 1700853 [https://doi.org/10.1183/13993003.00853-2017].

Chapter 2

Smoking and COPD: Endothelium-Related and Neuro-mediated Emphysema Mechanisms

Vera Nevzorova, Tatiana Brodskaya and Eugeny Gilifanov

Abstract

This chapter describes endothelium-related and neuro-mediated mechanisms of emphysema development in chronic obstructive pulmonary disease (COPD) and smoking on the basis of previously completed studies, literature data, and own researches. As components of neurogenic inflammation in the processes of tissue remodeling in emphysema, we describe the distribution and activity of the substance P, neurokinin-1 and its receptor, tissue metalloproteinases and their tissue inhibitors in the lungs during the entire experimental period, the modeling of COPD in rats with a smoking model. We also analyzed the content of neurokinin system markers, the localization, and markers of tissue metalloproteinases in human lung tissue structures. We have confidence that there is a special morpho-functional continuum of development of lower respiratory tract remodeling in response to chronic exposure to tobacco smoke and the development of inflammation in COPD. New data suggest that imbalance of neuro-mediated interactions, alteration of vasomotoric signaling mechanisms, secretion, mucociliary clearance, cytoprotection involving substance P-dependent components with impaired content, and development of dystopia of matrix metalloproteinases and their tissue inhibitors are involved in the initiation of morphological restructuring. Research in this direction should be continued to allow approaches to the development of preventive and therapeutic strategies for emphysema.

Keywords: COPD, smoking, emphysema, remodeling, neuro-mediated, endothelium, neurokinins, metalloproteinases

1. Introduction

Emphysema, or destruction of the gas-exchanging surfaces of the alveoli, is one of the typical manifestations of chronic obstructive pulmonary disease (COPD). Emphysema is a pathological term that is often used clinicaly, has great medical significance and describes only one of several structural abnormalities present in patients [1]. Many previous definitions of COPD have emphasized the terms "emphysema" and "chronic bronchitis," which are not included in the definition used in the last GOLD report. In GOLD 2018, COPD was defined as a common, preventable, and treatable disease that is characterized by persistent respiratory symptoms and airflow limitation that is due to airway and/or alveolar abnormalities usually caused by significant exposure to noxious particles or gases [1]. It was mentioned that chronic respiratory symptoms also exist in individuals with normal spirometry and a significant number of smokers without airflow limitation have structural evidence of lung disease manifested by the varying presence of emphysema, airway wall thickening, and gas trapping [2–4]. Really, smoking is a major risk factor for COPD, and it plays an important role in lung tissue destruction development. Some experiments prove that aggressive pollutants of tobacco smoke (benzopyrene, peroxynitrite, acrolein, cyanides, peroxides, etc.) can cause direct damage to endothelial cells due to expression of adhesion molecules on their surface and intensification of lipid peroxidation [2, 5–7]. But the main underlying cause of structural changes is chronic inflammation, which is confirmed by numerous studies [1, 4–6]. Even in mild COPD, or in smokers susceptible to emphysema [7, 8], there are significant abnormalities in pulmonary microvascular blood flow that worsen with disease progression [9].

It was proven that vascular endothelium actively participates in inflammatory reactions in COPD [10–13]. It was a systemized data about cigarette smoke as an endothelial toxin and activator [14]. Endothelium is one of the direct participants of development and maintenance of chronic inflammation. Oxidized lipoproteins in the tunica intima of the vessel work as attractants for chemotaxis of leukocytes and monocytes that start to produce pro-inflammatory cytokines in big amounts. These processes trigger systemic inflammatory response that leads to irreversible thickening of the vessel walls and deterioration of their mechanical properties. Chronic exposure to tobacco smoke and the products of combustion of tobacco lead to chronic system inflammatory reaction, oxidative stress, endothelial dysfunction, and morphofunctional damage of target organs. Nowadays the connection between endothelium-related mechanisms and emphysema forming, and progression in COPD is well known. Recent studies are approaching the description of the neuro-mediated mechanisms of emphysema development in COPD.

In this chapter we have analyzed data from researchers and shared our own research on the study of endothelium and the neuro-mediated mechanisms of emphysema development in COPD and smoking.

2. Endothelium-related and neuro-mediated mechanisms of emphysema development in COPD and smoking: research data

The participation of endothelial dysfunction and injury in emphysema development in COPD has been described since 2000 and early [15, 16]. And the interest of researchers to the problem of the involvement of the endothelium in the pathogenesis of COPD has not decreased over the past decades. So, for the request "endothelium + emphysema" (in the title and/or abstract), the well-known online resource of the library PubMed offers 117 publications, of which 23 after 2015. For the request "endothelium + COPD," it offers 335 publications, of which 72 after 2015, and for the request "endothelium + smoking," it offers 1859 publications, of which 188 after 2015. This indicates the relevance of this area of research and demonstrates the hopes of researchers finding new opportunities for therapeutic and prophylactic effects on this relationship in the pathogenesis of tobacco-related lesions, COPD, and emphysema [17–23].

All disorders begin with local and systemic inflammation, hypoxia and oxidative stress, and lead to an imbalance of proteases-antiproteases, loss of recovery and destruction of lung tissue. Activation and dysfunction of the endothelium involves, first of all, imbalance of the endothelium and its associated mechanisms, which are due to the following disorders in the pathogenesis of COPD [4]. Separately, we would like to pay attention on some endothelium-dependent factors.

Prolonged damage to endotheliocytes by aggression factors (persistent inflammation, hypoxia, oxidative stress, an imbalance in the protease-antiprotease system, etc.) leads to their death and anatomical reduction of the capillary bed, which is a component of emphysematous lung changes. Pathobiology of small vessels in COPD, in addition to inflammatory and hypercoagulative changes, is characterized by intimal thickening, arteriole muscularization, a decrease in the number of capillaries, and a decrease in blood vessels [13, 15]. Delivering a VEGF receptor (VEGFR) antagonist to rats led rapidly to air space enlargement and pruning of the pulmonary arterial tree [23, 24]. VEGF is a trophic factor that is crucial for the survival of endothelial cells. The experiment demonstrated that prolonged blockade of VEGF receptors leads to apoptosis of septal endothelial cells and emphysema [16, 25]. Subsequent studies of emphysematous lungs confirmed that COPD patients have decreased lung levels of VEGF, reduced expression of VEGFR in pulmonary endothelial cells and apoptotic alveolar septal cells, and reduced expression of hypoxia-inducible factor-1α (HIF-1α), a transcription factor that drives the expression of genes involved in endothelial function including VEGFRs [26, 27]. It has been shown that along with the progression of emphysema, degenerative changes in the walls of the aorta develop, including its dilatation and aneurysmatization [28, 29]. These facts indicate that among other circumstances, an important role in the pathogenesis of emphysema belongs to endotheliocytes and VEGF. Moreover, it has been described that the presence of emphysema in patients with COPD is associated with a reduced content of circulated endothelial cells, an endothelial repair factor [11, 30].

Endothelial dysfunction and damage are also caused by the acute effects of cigarette smoke long before the development of emphysema in animal models. Brief exposure of mice to cigarette smoke exacerbates lipopolysaccharide- and *Pseudomonas aeruginosa*-induced acute lung injury in vivo, and cigarette smoke extract increases the permeability of endothelial monolayers in vitro [14, 27]. Moreover, a recent study identified cigarette smoke-induced apoptosis of endothelial cells in the lungs of mice exposed chronically to cigarette smoke and COPD patients [11]. Thus, data from both animal models of COPD and COPD patients and controls support the hypothesis that endothelial dysfunction and injury are key processes in the pathogenesis of emphysema.

In **Table 1** we composed information on key endothelium-related agents that take into account the mechanisms of emphysema development in COPD, well described previously [4, 10–13, 18–20, 22, 23, 26, 27].

The mechanisms of the inclusion of neurokinins and related substances in neurogenic inflammation and destruction at different stages of COPD are much less known. Moreover, in recent studies, descriptions of the neuro-mediated mechanisms for the development of emphysema in COPD and smoking have become recognized.

It is known that tobacco smoke is a powerful inducer of the destruction of the respiratory epithelium throughout, followed by its morphofunctional remodeling [4, 31, 32]. Initiation of cell and tissue injury processes in prolonged exposure to smoking can take place due to excess release of neurotransmitters from sensitive afferent nerve fibers of the nervous vagus system. A large proportion (75%) of such fibers belong to the type of nonmyelinated or C-fibers, the sources of which are small neurons of the knotted and jugular ganglia, which synthesize neuropeptide transmitters or neurokinins (such as substance P (SP), a peptide genetically related to calcitonin (CGRP) and neurokinin (A)) [33, 34]. Afferent influences are primarily aimed at maintaining the structural and functional homeostasis of the respiratory system by stimulating the secretion of mucus from the submucous

Components	Origin, localization	Physiological effects and potential role at pathogenesis emphysema in COPD
Nitric oxide (NO)	In main, endothelial cells and other cells	Vasorelaxation, vasoprotection, anti-inflammatory, anti-adhesion, reparation. Endothelin antagonist
Endothelinum-1 (ET-1)	Endothelial cells, bronchial epithelium, alveolar macrophages	Activates receptors on smooth cells, encouraging stable vasoconstriction and increase of endothelium adhesively
sPECAM-1	Endothelial cells, lymphocytes, platelets, macrophages, granulocytes, T/NK-cell megakaryocytes, fibroblasts, osteoclasts	Plays a basic role in lymphocyte adhesion to vascular wall with followed effects
Selectins: E-selectin (CD62E), P-selectin (CD62P), L-selectin (CD62L)	Activated endothelial cells	Regulation of leukocyte adhesion (strengthens the capacity to migration, leukocyte adhesion to activated endothelium in inflammation)
Thrombomodulin (CD141)	Endothelial cells	Interacts with thrombin, activates protein C, acts as anticoagulant across activation factors fVa, fVIIIa, fXa, and fXIIIa
Circulated endothelial cells	Endothelial cells from vascular wall, activated bone marrow	Can be as the factor of reparation according to inflammatory processes and as the factor of injury to the endothelium and other tissues due to activated phenotype
Vascular endothelial growth factor (VEGF)	Endothelial cells	Main inductor of angiogenesis, VEGF, provides their effects across receptors' endothelial cell and expression of VEGF regulated by hypoxia, chronic inflammation, hypercoagulation, etc. In chronic processes, function can be an imperfect character Stimulates apoptosis and phagocytosis and promotes development of emphysema
Neutrophil elastase (catepsin G, proteinase 3)	Neutrophils, monocytes, T lymphocytes, endothelial cells, vascular smooth muscles cells	Decreases migration of T lymphocytes and neutrophil to inflammation area, factor of decelerating of phagocytosis. Function from protection to damaging. Can cause damage to tissues, development of emphysema, and mucus hypersecretion Involved in normal degradation of matrix proteins elastin, collagen, fibronectin, laminin, and proteoglycans
Matrix metalloproteinases (MMP-1, MMP-2, MMP-9)	Endothelial cells, macrophages, neutrophils, monocytes, fibroblasts, keratinocytes, osteoblasts	Contributes to release TNF-α from macrophages, that results to neutrophils recruiting and production neutrophil elastase, that leads to damage tissues, development emphysema. Involved in degradation of type IV collagen, fibronectin, and elastin

Table 1.
Endothelium-related Components of emphysema development in COPD and smoking [4, 10–13, 18–20, 22, 23, 26, 27].

glands and goblet cells, contractility of smooth muscles, vascular permeability, modulation of immune cascades, etc. [34–36]. It is known that afferent fibers (C-fibers) are extremely sensitive to the effects of irritants that make up tobacco smoke [37]. In a situation of prolonged and/or intense stimulation of sensory

Agents	Origin, localization	Physiological effects and potential role in emphysema pathogenesis in COPD	References
Neurokinins Substance P (SP)	Sensitive nerve endings. SP receptors on respiratory and glandular epithelial cells and endothelial cells. Neurokinin receptor-1 affixed to SP is found in submucous glands, and SP release from nociceptive nerves is responsible for secretion of glands	Belongs to the family of tachykinins, sensory peptides. Induces vasodilation and transudation of blood plasma in the respiratory tract. Induces chemotaxis of monocytes, neutrophils, and eosinophils and stimulates macrophages to produce mediators of inflammation and neutrophil elastase. Powerful mast cell stimulator, causing their degranulation. Sources and release of histamine and cytokine synthesis (IL-6). Takes part in neurogenic inflammation when stimulating the production of IgA from B lymphocytes and cytokines from T-helper cells. Enhances the release of acetylcholine from the postganglionic cholinergic nerves of the respiratory tract It causes smooth muscle contraction, secretion of submucous glands, vasodilation, and increased vascular permeability. Tobacco smoking inhibits the activity of the enzyme endopeptidase, which enhances the activity of SP	[40, 45, 48, 49]
Neurokinins Neurokinin A	The highest density in the nerve fibers around the arteries. Tachykinin receptor subtypes NK1, NK2, and NK3	Belongs to the family of tachykinins, sensory peptides. Contraction of smooth muscles; secretion of submucous glands; vasodilation; increased vascular permeability; stimulation of cholinergic nerves, mast cells, B and T lymphocytes, and macrophages; eosinophil chemoattraction; and adhesion of neutrophils in the vessels of the respiratory tract with activation following	[44, 50, 51]
Neuropeptide -γ	It is produced in some of the upper cervical ganglia and the bodies of the main palatine cells Sympathetic nerves contain either norepinephrine or norepinephrine and neuropeptide Y	Reduces the frequency of vibrations of ciliary cells induced by cholinergic nerves, providing an inhibitory effect on these nerves Sympathetic reflexes cause vasoconstriction and can also stimulate the secretion of certain glands in the trachea and bronchi	[38, 39, 48]
Receptor NK1	NK1 tachykinin receptor mRNA is found in the pulmonary arteries, veins, and human bronchi, in the endothelium of the veins and arteries, and in the smooth muscles of the bronchi, as well as in lymphocytes, macrophages, and mastocytes	The tachykinin receptor NK1, with the highest affinity for SP. SP, in turn, is a powerful mast cell stimulator, causing their degranulation, and induces the chemotaxis of monocytes, neutrophils, eosinophils, and stimulates macrophages to produce inflammatory mediators and neutrophilic elastase	[40, 42, 45]

Agents	Origin, localization	Physiological effects and potential role in emphysema pathogenesis in COPD	References
Receptor NK2 Receptor NK3	NK2 receptor mRNA is abundantly expressed in the human bronchi and weakly in the pulmonary veins and arteries NK3 tachykinin receptor mRNA is found in the pulmonary arteries, veins, and human bronchi	The tachykinin receptor NK2, with the highest affinity for neurokinin A. Tachykinin receptor NK3, with the highest affinity for neurokinin B The release of histamine from mouse mast cells is mediated through tachykinin NK2 receptors	[40, 42, 45, 52]

Table 2.
Potential neuro-mediated mechanisms of emphysema development in COPD and tobacco smoking.

fibers, excessive release of neuropeptide mediator is accompanied by a number of plastic and destructive processes due to a cascade of pathological reactions of neurogenic inflammation [38, 39]. In addition to substance P of neuronal origin, neuropeptides from cells of the immune system—eosinophils, basophils, monocytes, macrophages and lymphocytes—join the realization of neurogenic inflammation [38, 40, 41]. The obtained data indicate the role of the disturbance of the activity of the neurokinin system in the development and maintenance of morphofunctional changes in the pathology of the respiratory tract associated with smoking [42–46]. Chronic exposure to cigarette smoke has been shown to increase SP expression in neurons of the central nervous system [35–37] and simultaneously inhibits the activity of enzymes that metabolize neurokinins [39, 40, 43]. According to experimental study, even low concentrations of cigarette smoke significantly reduce the topical activity of neuronal endopeptidase and increase the concentration of CP in the respiratory tract [35]. The contribution of excessive sensitivity of NK1 receptors in the airways to the development of bronchoconstriction under the influence of tobacco smoke irritants and/or during bronchial asthma has been proven [42, 43, 47]. At the same time, the components and mechanisms of neurogenic inflammation in the development of emphysema associated with prolonged exposure to tobacco smoke are poor and fragmentary in the literature.

In **Table 2** we have tried to compose information about potential neuro-mediated mechanisms of emphysema development in COPD and tobacco smoking.

3. Mechanisms of neurogenic inflammation in the tissue remodeling processes in emphysema: own researches

3.1 Study of the neurogenic inflammation mechanisms in the emphysema formation in the experiment

To study the contribution of the components of neurogenic inflammation to the processes of tissue remodeling in pulmonary emphysema associated with smoking, an experimental model of long-term tobacco smoking in vivo in rats was reproduced. The experiment was performed in appliance with the model D. According to Zheng [53] in our own modification [54], the duration of exposure to tobacco smoke in terms of human life is 12 years. The features of the

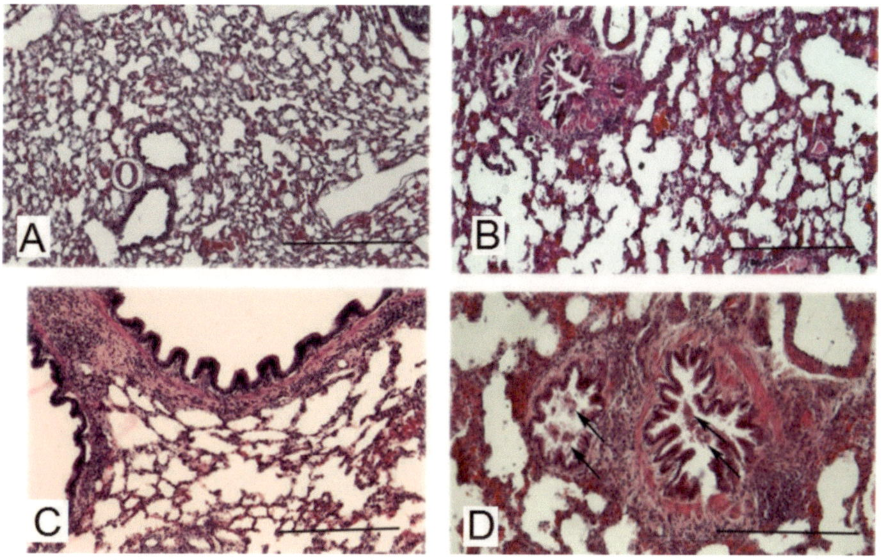

Figure 1.
The lung (A, B) and bronchi (C, D) of animals in the control group (A, C) and rats with the DTC model (B, D). Coloring: hematoxylin-eosin. Scale: A, B (500 microns); C, D (100 microns).

distribution and activity of SP, NK1, MMP-2, MMP-9, and TIMP-2 in the tissues of the mucous membrane of the lungs were performed using the immunoperoxidase method on cryostat sections of 15 μm in thickness according to standard methods. The following primary antibodies were used: anti-SP (Abcam, ab 14184, 1:200, CIIIA), anti-NK1 (Chemicon AB 5060, 1:500, USA), anti-MMP2 (rabbit polyclonal, ThermoScientific), anti-MMP9 (rabbit polyclonal, ThermoScientific, rb-9234-p, 1:200), anti-TIMP2 (rabbit polyclonal, Abcam, ab61224, 1:100), secondary biotinylated antibodies (ThermoScientific, 1:200), streptavidin peroxidase (ThermoScientific), and chromogen (Peroxidase Substrate Kit, VectorNovaRED, SK-4800). Morphological studies were performed in the laboratory of the Pacific State Medical University.

The results of morphological studies of the bronchopulmonary system of rats in the control group and with the model of long-term tobacco smoking are presented in **Figure 1**.

Morphological changes in the lungs of rats with a long-term tobacco smoking model are focal. Over the entire area of the slice of the lungs, there are fields with pronounced emphysematous changes, accompanied by loss of the integrity of the alveoli and the formation of large emphysematous expansions, an increase in the thickness of the interalveolar septa (**Figure 1B, D**). In other parts of the lung parenchyma, there are signs of swelling and/or hemorrhagic impregnation in peribronchial spaces. Cellular composition contains cells of immune inflammation—plasma cells, lymphocytes, and macrophages.

The distribution of the components of the neurokinin system of rats obtained by morphological examination of the bronchi and lungs coincides with the previously described data [55] and is shown in **Figure 2**. Nerve fibers secreting SP are presented in the subepithelial zones of the bronchi (**Figure 2A**); their penetration is recorded in the epithelial layer (**Figure 2B**), pulmonary parenchyma (**Figure 2D**), and adventitia of pulmonary vessels (**Figure 2E**).

The morphometry of the components of the neurokinin system in the bronchopulmonary system of rats was compared with the model of long-term tobacco smoking and control animals (**Table 3**).

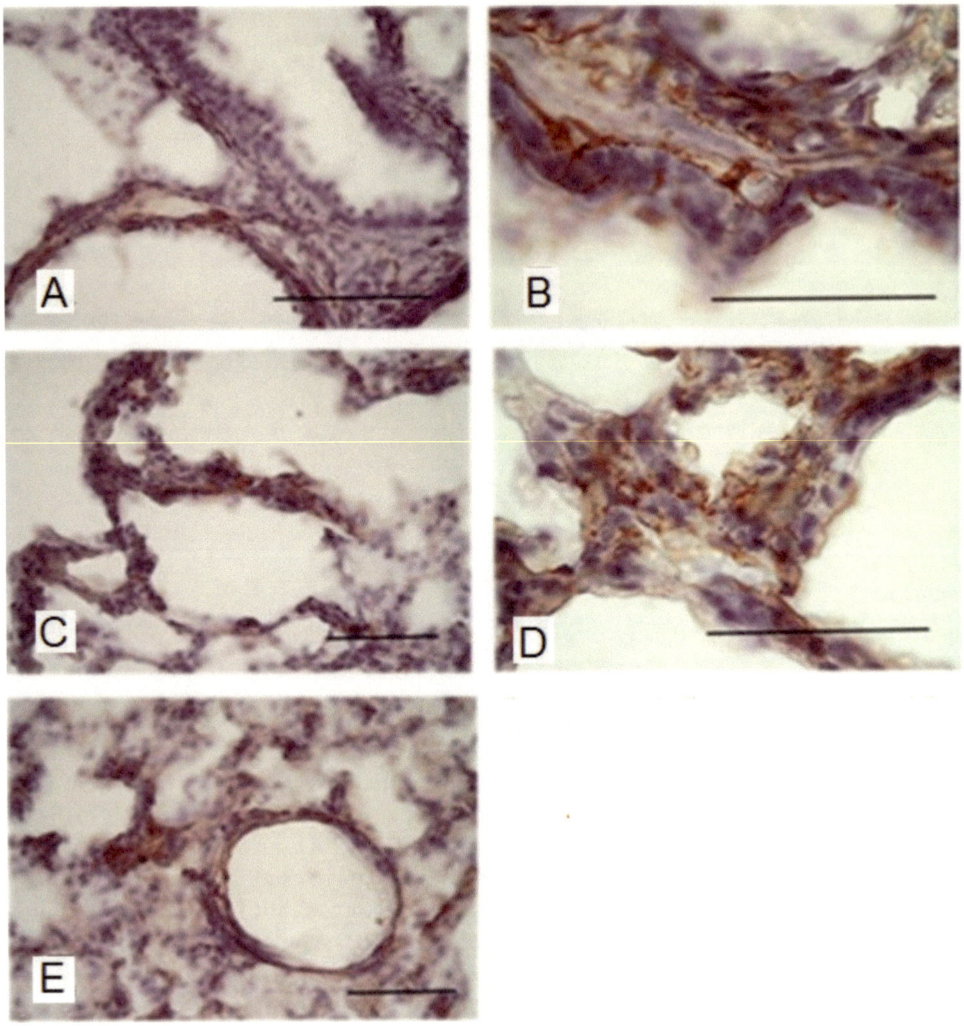

Figure 2.
Distribution of SP- and NK1-reactive structures in the bronchopulmonary system of rats. Coloring: immunoperoxidase reaction on SP; repainting, hematoxylin-eosin. Scale: A, 100 microns; B–E, 50 microns.

The content of SP-containing fibers and NK1-positive structures in the control group and in the model of long-term tobacco smoking shows an ambiguous pattern. An increase in the distribution area of SP-immunopositive nerve fibers in the lungs and bronchi of experimental animals was found to be 10.7 and 9.4%, respectively, compared with the control group. The most significant increase in fiber density was observed in the adventitia of pulmonary parenchyma vessels compared with other structures. Being a vasodilator, substance P increases vascular permeability and promotes adhesion and penetration of leukocytes into the surrounding tissues for the realization of local immune reactions involved in the development of destructive processes in the pulmonary parenchyma. Regarding NK1-positive elements, it should be noted that there is no change in their content in the lung tissue and a moderate increase in the density in the bronchial wall against the background of a decrease in the total number and NK1-immunoreactive tissue basophils. Obviously, substance P plays a key role in the implementation of neurogenic inflammation processes in chronic exposure to tobacco smoke. The established pattern of changes in NK1-positive structures can be explained by the ability of SP to cause mast cell degranulation and NK1 receptor-dependent release of histamine and serotonin involved in local inflammatory answer.

Indicator	Bronchi		Lungs	
	Control	Experiment (long-term smoking model)	Control	Experiment (long-term smoking model)
SP distribution area (%)	5.11 ± 0.36	5.59 ± 0.14*	4.60 ± 0.29	5.10 ± 0.34*
NK1 distribution area (%)	0.27 ± 0.03	0.31 ± 0.03*	0.16 ± 0.016	0.16 ± 0.02
NK1-positive mast cells (in 1 mm^3 of the tissue)			92.68 ± 19.26	76.39 ± 15.74*
General population of tissue basophils (in 1 mm^3 of the tissue)			129.53 ± 19.64	106.93 ± 7.64*

*The differences are significant with $p < 0.05$.

Table 3.
Morphometric characteristics of SP- and NK1-immunoreactive structures in the bronchopulmonary system of rats.

One of the leading stimulators of the synthesis of substance P in the model of long-term tobacco smoking is hypoxia which changes the humoral regulation of blood flow [55]. SP can adjust the change in vessel diameter at the unchanged vascular wall using an axon reflex for adequate blood flow at a given point in time. However, when the architectonics of the vascular wall changes, the SP loses its function as a regulator and can participate in both excessive vasodilation and paradoxical vasoconstriction.

In the development of the structural remodeling of the respiratory system, there are several morphological phenomena that accompany this process and are the basis for the development of reversible and irreversible morphofunctional changes. These include thinning of the epithelial layer, development of subepithelial fibrosis, an increase in smooth muscle thickness, an increase in the number and/or size of the submucosal glands, and the activation of angiogenesis processes [56]. In the pathogenesis of the changes taking place, great importance is attached to the activity of the enzymes of the extracellular matrix, which ensure the degradation of its interstitial proteins. Modern advances in proteomics have shown that for normal development, physiological renewal, restoration of healthy tissues, and the formation of pathological changes in tissue morphology, two groups of proteins are leading—MMPs and their tissue inhibitors [57, 58]. MMPs are a family of 20 zinc and calcium-dependent endopeptidases capable of cleaving almost all components of the extracellular matrix of connective tissues [59]. The level of synthesis and secretion of MMP into the extracellular space is regulated by transcription factors, and their proteolytic activity depends on the chemical transformations of the enzyme molecule in the interstitial space. As a result, either activation of the proenzymes or inhibition of their active forms can be observed. Depending on the type of protein metabolized, MMP can be divided into collagenases (MMP-1, MMP-8, and MMP-13), gelatinase (MMP-2 and MMP-9), stromalins (MMP-3 and MMP-10), etc. [60, 61]. In mammals there are four known TIMPs that inhibit all MMPs in a 1:1 ratio by strong covalent bonding [62]. It is believed that the balance of proteolytic and antiproteolytic mechanisms maintained in different tissues and organs is carried out by a specific set of intercellular matrix enzymes and their inhibitors [59, 63]. On the other hand, each process has a specific set of depressed matrix proteolytic enzymes. In this regard, great prospects in creating targeted therapy for many pathological processes are associated with the determination of the tissue specificity of the enzymes of the extracellular matrix and the identification of patterns of changes in their activity during the development of pathology.

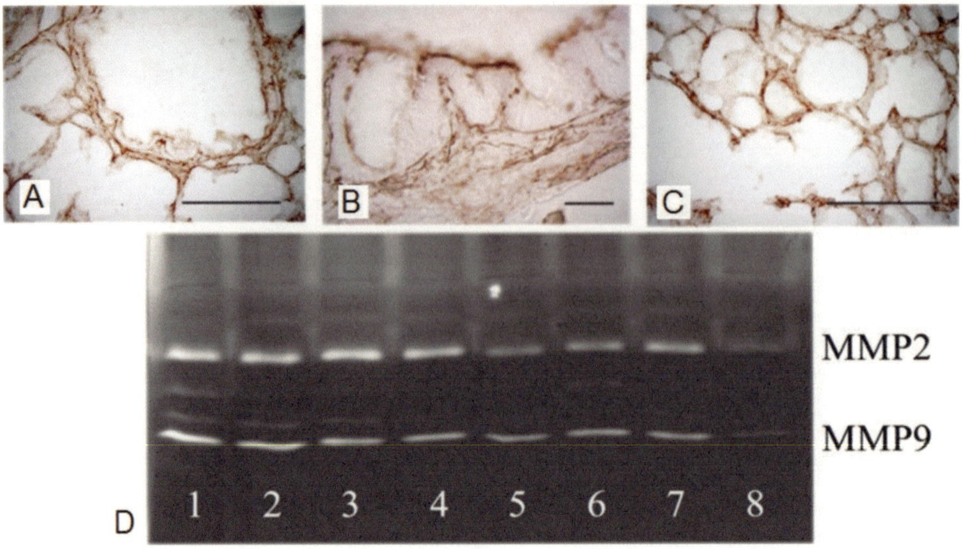

Figure 3.
Immunohistochemical (A–C) and biochemical determination of MMP in the bronchopulmonary system of rats with a model of long-term tobacco smoking. Coloring—immunohistochemical reaction to MMP-2 and MMP-9. Scale: A, B, B—50 µm. Localization of MMP-2 in the wall of the bronchus (A, B) and interalveolar septa (C). (D) Zymogram of MMP-2 and MMP-9. Lanes 1–4, lung homogenates of rats of the control group; lanes 5–8, lung homogenates of rats with a model of long-term tobacco smoking.

Indicators	Control	Experiment (long-term smoking model)	Control	Experiment (long-term smoking model)
	MMP-9		MMP-2	
Conventional density units	742689.75	450081.25*	367243.25	246414.75*
MMP-9/MMP-2	2.02 (control)		1.83 (experiment (long-term smoking model))	

The differences are significant with $p < 0.05$.

Table 4.
The contents of MMP-2 and MMP-9 in the homogenates of the lungs of rats.

A number of studies have shown the role of individual types of MMP in the development of nicotine-associated pathology of the lungs and bronchi [57, 58]. To clarify the role of the leading MMP—MMP9 related to the inducible form and MMP2—considered as a constitutive variant of the enzyme in the development of pulmonary emphysema associated with long-term smoking, we studied the immunohistochemical and biochemical content of enzymes in the tissues and homogenates of rats with long-term smoking patterns (**Figure 3**).

In the bronchopulmonary system of rats, prolonged exposure to tobacco smoke is accompanied by ambiguous dynamics of the content of matrix metalloproteinases and their inhibitors. Normally, the activity of MMP-2 and MMP-9 is recorded in the cytoplasm and processes of bronchial and pulmonary fibroblasts, which form a thin MMP-positive strip in the lamina propria of the bronchial mucosa (**Figure 3A, B**) and in the interalveolar septa (**Figure 3C**). In the lungs and bronchi of rats with the long-term tobacco smoking model, a marked decrease in the immunohistochemical activity of MMP-2 and MMP-9 was observed. At the same time, in the acute phase of the experiment, the number and intensity of coloring of immunopositive structures on MMP-2 and MMP-9 are higher than in the control group. According to the quantitative

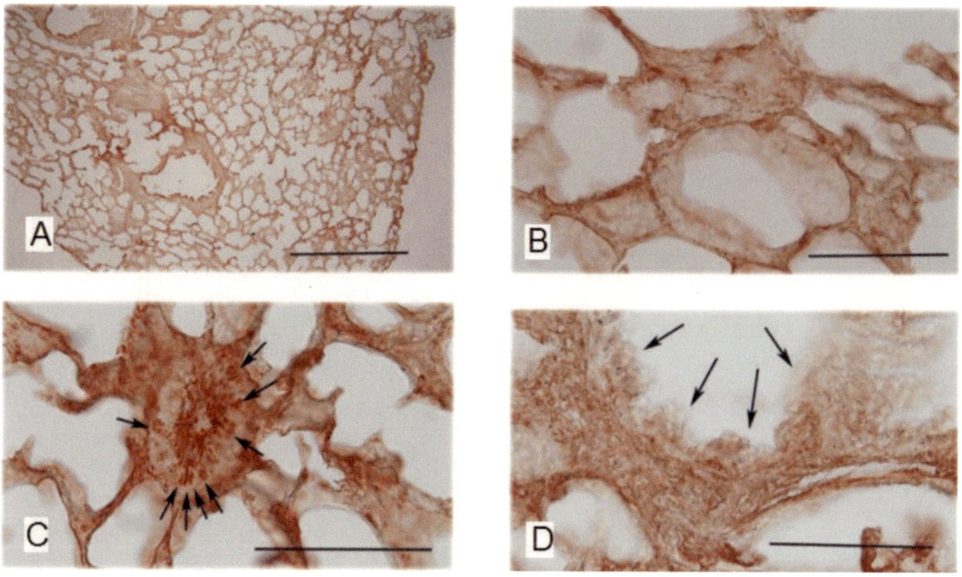

Figure 4.
The distribution of the content of TIMP-2 in the lungs of rats of the control (A–C) and with the model of long-term tobacco smoking (D) groups. Coloring—immunohistochemical reaction to TIMP-2. Scale A, 100 microns; GD, 50 microns. A total enzyme content in the tissues of the bronchopulmonary system. B-TIMP-2-positive fibroblasts of the interalveolar septa. B-content of the enzyme in the epithelial cells of the small bronchus (indicated by arrows). G-reduction of the enzyme content in epithelial cells of the bronchus of rats with a model of prolonged smoking (indicated by arrows).

determination of enzymes in the homogenates of lung tissue (**Figure 3D**, **Table 4**), the resulting trend is confirmed. That is, with the development of pulmonary emphysema associated with prolonged smoking in the lung tissue, the content of both MMPs decreases evenly.

An analysis of the immunohistochemical composition of the tissue inhibitor of both MMP and TIMP-2 showed a marked decrease in its representation in the structures of the bronchopulmonary system of animals on a model of long-term smoking (**Figure 4**).

In intact animals, the enzyme localization occurs in the respiratory epithelial cells of the bronchial membrane (**Figure 4C**, indicated by arrows) and fibroblasts of the interalveolar septa (**Figure 4B**). In animals of the main group, the overall intensity of immunohistochemical staining of lung tissue decreases, and at high magnifications of the microscope, it is possible to fix a significant depression of the color or complete disappearance of the enzyme content in the epithelial lining cells of the bronchi and lung parenchyma tissue (**Figure 4**, indicated by arrows).

According to the data obtained, the immunolocalization of MMP-2, MMP-9, and TIMP-2 repeats the basic pattern of distribution of pro-inflammatory cells and coincides with the foci of the most noticeable rearrangements of the connective tissue of the bronchi and the pulmonary parenchyma. In the acute phase of the experiment, the activity of the markers is significantly higher compared to the control; after 6 months of exposure to smoke, there is a decrease of the proteolytic activity and at the same time the processes of its inhibition.

3.2 Study of the neurogenic inflammation mechanisms of the emphysema formation in humans

In addition to studying the processes of neurogenic inflammation and the contribution of matrix metalloproteinases to the development of emphysema in the

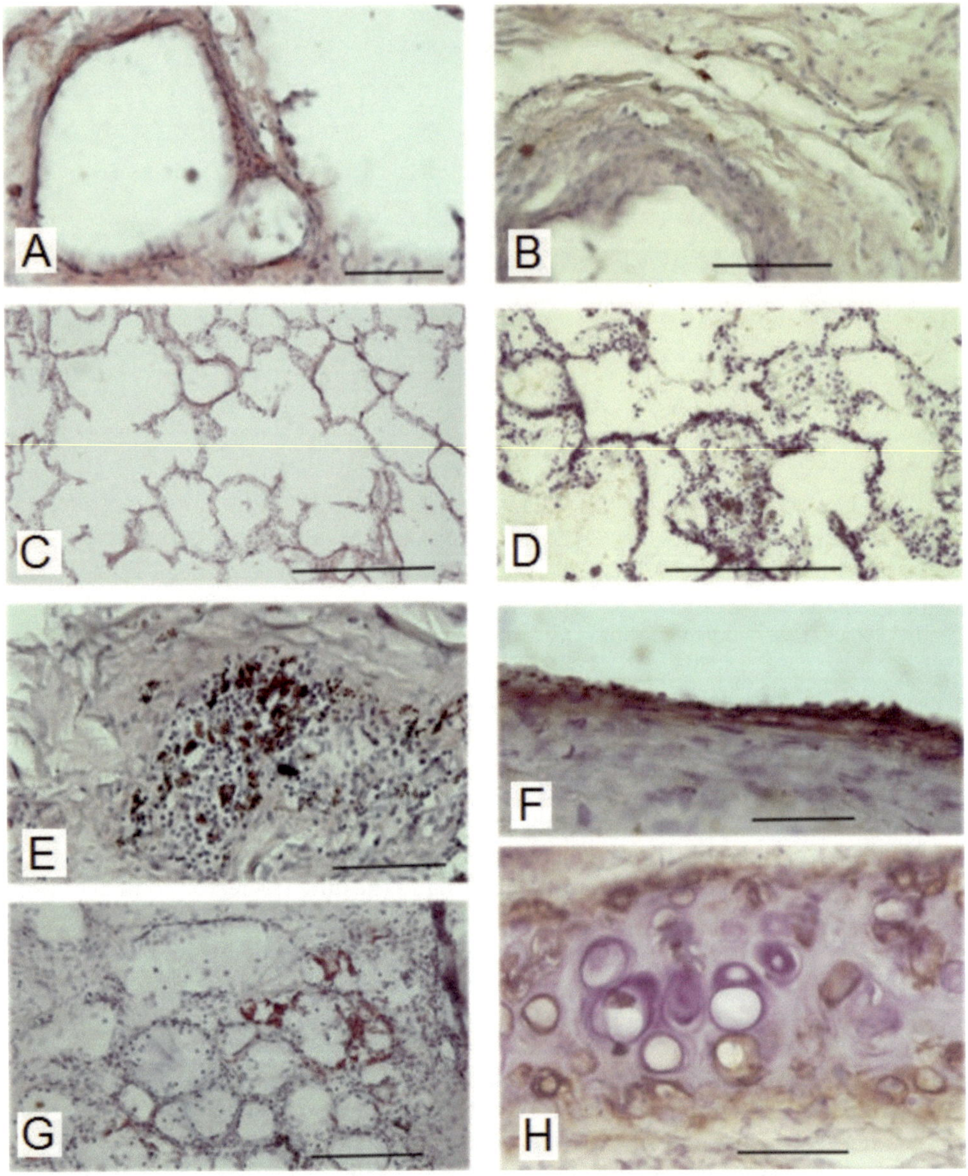

Figure 5.
Distribution of the content of SP (A, C, E, G) and NK1 (B, D, F, H) in the bronchopulmonary system in persons with emphysema. Coloring: immunohistochemical reaction to SP and NK1, stained with hematoxylin. Scale: A, B, E, G (50 microns); C, D (100 microns); and F, H (20 microns). Nerve fibers innervating the wall of the bronchus (A) and interalveolar partitions (C). Localization of SP-positive macrophages in peribronchial infiltrates (E). SP-positive glandulocytes of the bronchial glands (G). Localization of neurokinin receptors on the surface of peribronchial macrophages (B), dust macrophages (D), vascular endothelial cells (F), and chondrocytes of the fibrocartilage membrane of the bronchi (H).

experiment, we analyzed the content of neurokinin system markers, the localization, and the content of MMP-2, MMP-9, and TIMP-2 in human lung tissue structures. Morphological studies of autopsy material were performed on 12 individuals aged 51–65 years and 3 women and 9 men, average age 61.5 ± 4.14 years, who died a sudden death outside the hospital. The long-term history of tobacco smoking was clarified from the close relatives and on the basis of the data of the outpatient card. Features of the distribution and activity of SP, NK1, MMP-9, and TIMP-2, in lung tissues were investigated using the immunoperoxidase method on cryostat sections of 15 μm in thickness according to the standard procedure using the primary antibody line described above.

In lung tissue and bronchial wall of patients with pulmonary emphysema, positive SP immunoreactivity is found mainly in the nerve fibers (**Figure 5**). More common are single conductors having a uniform ribbonlike course and numerous varicose thickenings. With a successful coincidence of the cut plane with the spatial geometry of the fibers, it is possible to observe beams extending 300–500 μm. Fibers penetrate through the walls of the bronchi of medium and small caliber, spread around the perimeter of the submucosa (**Figure 5A, B**). In the interstitial tissue, lightweight fibers have a diameter of 0.5–1 microns, and sometimes they are grouped into clusters with the formation of numerous terminals. Probably, the latter are areas of the most dense accumulation of neuromuscular and glandular contacts. The morphological characteristics of the colored conductors allow them to be treated as mixed (afferent and motor) fibers. High SP expression is also detected in peribronchial leukocyte infiltrates (**Figure 5D**). Here, high immunoreactivity is observed for neurokinin receptors of type 1 (**Figure 5B, D**). The preferential localization of the NK1 surface of the membranes of the secretory epithelial cells of the bronchial glands, alveolar and stromal macrophages, microvascular endothelial cells, and elements of the fibrocartilage membrane (**Figure 5B, D, E, H**) should be emphasized.

Prolonged pathological effects of tobacco combustion products entail the formation of structural changes with the active involvement of the neurokinin innervation apparatus localized in the mucous membranes of the respiratory system. The increase in the number of macrophage cells and NK1-positive macrophages, and the direct interaction between them and afferent fibers, through terminals, suggests the involvement of sensory nerve fibers in the regulation of local immune,

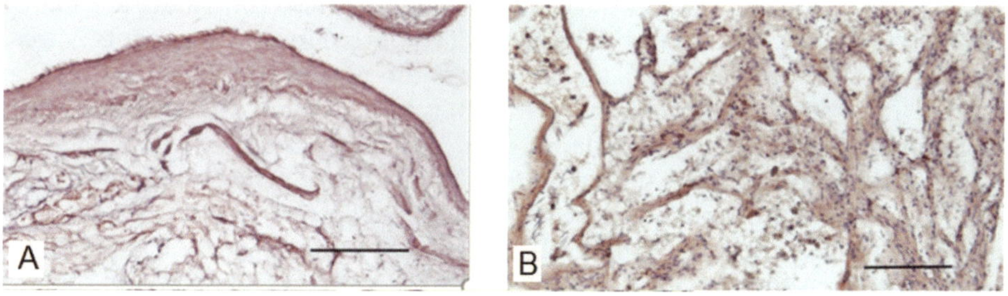

Figure 6.
Localization of MMP-9 in the lungs (A, B) of a person. Coloring: immunohistochemical reaction to MMP-9, stained with hematoxylin. Scale: A (50 microns); B (100 microns).

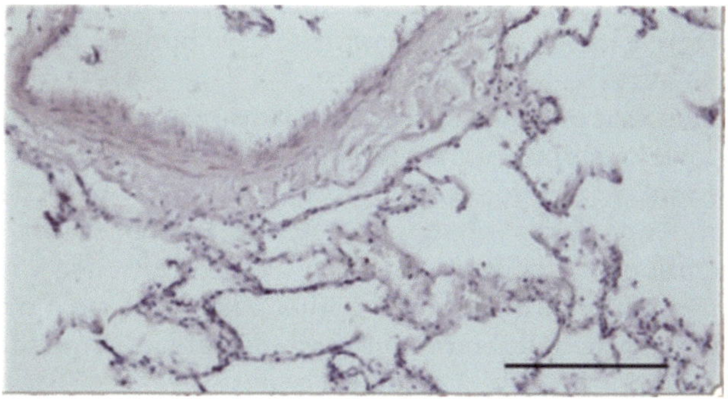

Figure 7.
Localization of TIMP-2 pulmonary parenchyma in individuals with emphysema. Coloring: immunohistochemical reaction to TIMP-2, stained with hematoxylin. Scale: 100 microns.

inflammatory, and destructive processes in the lung tissue during smoking-induced emphysema.

In contrast to the experimental data, in individuals with long periods of smoking and emphysema, there is an increase in the immunohistochemical density of MMP-9 in the pulmonary parenchyma (**Figure 6**), while TIMP-2 is practically undetermined (**Figure** 7).

In this way, from the presented data of experimental modeling of emphysema associated with long-term smoking, as well as studies in people with pulmonary emphysema and long-term tobacco smoking experience, neurogenic inflammation takes an active part in the processes of remodeling of lung tissue. Markers of neuro-mediated inflammation activity are overexpression of SP-containing nerve fibers, the presence of NK-1-tagged macrophages, mast cell degranulation, and an immune-mediated pattern of inflammatory infiltrate. Pathomorphosis of pulmonary parenchyma destruction in nicotine-associated pulmonary emphysema is associated with dysregulation in the state of the family of matrix metalloproteinases. In the acute period of exposure to tobacco combustion products, overexpression of MMP-9 is observed with suppression of the activity of the tissue inhibitor TIMP-2, followed by depression of the tissue content of both MMP-2 and MMP-9 and an inhibitor of their activity TIMP-2. In individuals with pulmonary emphysema, the MMP-9 tissue pattern retains its excessive representation.

4. Conclusions and future directions

Results from human and animal studies indicate that endothelial dysfunction and injury contribute not only to the genesis and progression of pulmonary lesions in COPD (especially emphysema development) but may also contribute to some of the common comorbidities and systemic effects reported in COPD patients. Vascular endothelium initiates and modulates the main pathomorphic processes in COPD and smoking. In particular, endothelium activation is an important factor of initiation, development and persistence of inflammation, and vessel and tissue remodeling, in particular emphysema. It is not by chance that the relationship of emphysema of the lungs is described in violation of the mechanical properties of the aorta and excessive stiffness of other exponents' bloodstream [4, 6, 64]. At the basis of these pathological processes are common (genetically determined and pathologically determined) mechanisms associated with impaired collagen-elastin metabolism.

The latest studies are conducted in the direction of studying not simple, associated with the endothelium, but specific neuro-mediated mechanisms of emphysema development in COPD and smoking. Our studies presented in this chapter describe the study of the processes of neurogenic inflammation and the contribution of matrix metalloproteinases to the development of emphysema in the experiment and in humans.

We are confident that there is a special morphofunctional continuum in the development of lower respiratory tract remodeling in response to chronic exposure to tobacco smoke and the development of inflammation in COPD. New data suggest that imbalance of neuro-mediated interactions, alteration of vasomotoric signaling mechanisms, secretion, mucociliary clearance, cytoprotection involving substance P-dependent components with impaired content, and development of dystopia of matrix metalloproteinases and their tissue inhibitors are involved in the initiation of morphological restructuring. Future studies should also assess the extent to which endothelial dysfunction and injury, particularly neuro-mediated mechanisms, underlie emphysema in COPD and smoking as target to therapeutic and prophylactic impacts.

Conflict of interest

No any conflict of interests.

Acronyms and abbreviations

COPD	Chronic obstructive pulmonary disease
VEGF	Vascular endothelial growth factor
VEGFR	VEGF receptor
NO	Nitric oxide
ET-1	Endothelinum-1
sPECAM-1	Soluble platelet endothelial cell adhesion molecule
VEGF	Vascular endothelial growth factor
MMP	Matrix metalloproteinases
SP	Substance P

Author details

Vera Nevzorova, Tatiana Brodskaya* and Eugeny Gilifanov
Pacific State Medical University, Vladivostok, Russia

*Address all correspondence to: brodskaya@mail.ru

References

[1] Global Initiative for Chronic Obstructive Pulmonary Disease [Internet]. 2018. Available from: http://www.goldcopd.org

[2] Woodruff PG, Barr RG, Bleecker E, et al. Clinical significance of symptoms in smokers with preserved pulmonary function. The New England Journal of Medicine. 2016;**374**(19):1811-1821. DOI: 10.1056/NEJMoa1505971

[3] Regan EA, Lynch DA, Curran-Everett D, et al. Clinical and radiologic disease in smokers with normal spirometry. JAMA Internal Medicine. 2015;**175**(9):1539-1549. DOI: 10.1001/jamainternmed.2015.2735

[4] Nevzorova V, Brodskaya T, Zakharchuk N. Smocking, respiratory diseases and endothelial dysfunction. In: Lenasi H, editor. Endothelial Dysfunction: Old Concepts and New Challenges. London: IntechOpen; 2018. pp. 307-326. ISBN 978-953-51-5698-7. DOI: 10.5772/intechopen.73555

[5] Sakao S, Voelkel NF, Tatsumi K. The vascular bed in COPD: Pulmonary hypertension and pulmonary vascular alterations. European Respiratory Review. 2014;**23**(133):350-355. DOI: 10.1007/978-3-662-47178-4_14

[6] Brodskaya TA, Geltser BI, Nevzorova VA. Arterial Stiffness and Respiratory Deseases (Pathophysiological Mechanisms and Clinical Significance). Vladivostok: Dalnauka; 2008. 248 p. ISBN 978-5-8044-0928-0

[7] Alford SK, van Beek EJ, McLennan G, Hoffman EA. Heterogeneity of pulmonary perfusion as a mechanistic image-based phenotype in emphysema susceptible smokers. Proceedings of the National Academy of Sciences of the United States of America. 2010;**107**(16):7485-7490. DOI: 10.1073/pnas.0913880107

[8] Iyer KS, Newell JD Jr, Jin D, et al. Quantitative dual-energy computed tomography supports a vascular etiology of smoking-induced inflammatory lung disease. American Journal of Respiratory and Critical Care Medicine. 2016;**193**(6):652-661. DOI: 10.1164/rccm.201506-1196OC

[9] Peinado VI, Pizarro S, Barbera JA. Pulmonary vascular involvement in COPD. Chest. 2008;**134**(4):808-814. DOI: 10.1378/chest.08-0820

[10] Brodskaya TA, Nevzorova VA, Geltser BI, Motkina EV. Endothelial dysfunction and respiratory disease. Terapevticheskij Arkhiv. 2007;**79**(3): 76-84. PMID: 17526203

[11] Polverino BR, Celli CA. Owen COPD as an endothelial disorder: Endothelial injury linking lesions in the lungs and other organs? Pulmonary Circulation. 2018;**8**(1):2045894018758528. DOI: 10.1177/2045894018758528. PMID: 29468936

[12] Moro L, Pedone C, Scarlata S, et al. Endothelial dysfunction in chronic obstructive pulmonary disease. Angiology. 2008;**59**:357-364. DOI: 10.1177/0003319707306141

[13] Vukic DA, Ruzic A, Samarzija M, et al. Persistent endothelial dysfunction turns the frequent exacerbator COPD from respiratory disorder into a progressive pulmonary and systemic vascular disease. Medical Hypotheses. 2015;**84**:155-158. DOI: 10.1016/S2213-2600(17)30236-9

[14] Voelkel NF. Cigarette smoke is an endothelial cell toxin. American Journal of Respiratory and Critical Care Medicine. 2018;**197**:274. DOI: 10.1164/rccm.201706-1123LE

[15] Kasahara Y, Tuder RM, Taraseviciene-Stewart L, et al.

Inhibition of VEGF receptors causes lung cell apoptosis and emphysema. The Journal of Clinical Investigation. 2000;**106**:1311-1319. DOI: 10.1172/JCI10259

[16] Voelkel NF, Cool CD. Pulmonary vascular involvement in chronic obstructive pulmonary disease. The European Respiratory Journal Supplement. 2003;**46**:28s-32s. DOI: 10.1183/09031936.03.00000503. PMID: 14621104

[17] Huertas A, Guignabert C, Barberà JA, Bärtsch P, Bhattacharya J, et al. Pulmonary vascular endothelium: The orchestra conductor in respiratory diseases: Highlights from basic research to therapy. The European Respiratory Journal. 2018;**51**(4):1700745. DOI: 10.1183/13993003.00745-2017. PMID: 29545281

[18] Letsiou E, Bauer N. Endothelial extracellular vesicles in pulmonary function and disease. Current Topics in Membranes. 2018;**82**:197-256. DOI: 10.1016/bs.ctm.2018.09.002. PMID: 30360780

[19] Green CE, Turner AM. The role of the endothelium in asthma and chronic obstructive pulmonary disease (COPD). Respiratory Research. 2017;**18**(1):20. DOI: 10.1186/s12931-017-0505-1. PMID: 8100233

[20] García-Lucio J, Peinado VI, de Jover L, Del Pozo R, Blanco I, et al. Imbalance between endothelial damage and repair capacity in chronic obstructive pulmonary disease. PLoS One. 2018;**13**(4):e0195724. DOI: 10.1371/journal.pone.0195724. PMID: 29672621

[21] Lu Q, Gottlieb E, Rounds S. Effects of cigarette smoke on pulmonary endothelial cells. American Journal of Physiology Lung Cellular and Molecular Physiology. 2018;**314**(5):L743-L756. DOI: 10.1152/ajplung.00373.2017. PMID: 29351435

[22] Cui M, Cui R, Liu K, Dong JY, Imano H, et al. Associations of tobacco smoking with impaired endothelial function: The circulatory risk in communities study (CIRCS). Journal of Atherosclerosis and Thrombosis. 2018;**25**(9):836-845. DOI: 10.5551/jat.42150. PMID: 29415955

[23] Skurikhin EG, Krupin VA, Pershina OV, Pan ES, Ermolaeva LA, et al. Endothelial progenitor cells and Notch-1 signaling as markers of alveolar endothelium regeneration in pulmonary emphysema. Bulletin of Experimental Biology and Medicine. 2018;**166**(2): 201-206. DOI: 10.1007/s10517-018-4314-4. PMID: 30488216

[24] Truong TM, Li H, Dhapare S, Desai UR, Voelkel NF, Sakagami M. Sulfated dehydropolymer of caffeic acid: In vitro anti-lung cell death activity and in vivo intervention in emphysema induced by VEGF receptor blockade. Pulmonary Pharmacology & Therapeutics. 2017;**45**:181-190. DOI: 10.1016/j.pupt.2017.06.007

[25] Tuder RM, Zhen L, Cho CY, et al. Oxidative stress and apoptosis interact and cause emphysema due to vascular endothelial growth factor receptor blockade. American Journal of Respiratory Cell and Molecular Biology. 2003;**29**(1):88-97. DOI: 10.1165/rcmb.2002-0228OC

[26] Kasahara Y, Tuder RM, Cool CD, et al. Endothelial cell death and decreased expression of vascular endothelial growth factor and vascular endothelial growth factor receptor 2 in emphysema. American Journal of Respiratory and Critical Care Medicine. 2001;**163**: 737-744. DOI: 10.1164/ajrccm.163.3.2002117

[27] Yasuo M, Mizuno S, Kraskauskas D, et al. Hypoxia inducible factor-1alpha in human emphysema lung tissue. The European Respiratory

Journal. 2011;**37**:775-783. DOI: 10.1183/09031936.00022910

[28] Buckley C, Wyble CW, Borhani M, et al. Accelerated enlargement of experimental abdominal aortic aneurysms in a mouse model of chronic cigarette smoke exposure. Journal of the American College of Surgeons. 2004;**199**(6):896-903. DOI: 10.1016/j.jamcollsurg.2004.08.010

[29] Takagi H, Umemoto TJ. How cigarette smoke accelerates abdominal aortic aneurysm. American College of Surgeons. 2005;**201**(1):149-150. DOI: 10.1016/j.jamcollsurg.2005.03.011. PMID: 15978458

[30] Lee JH. Decreased number of circulating endothelial progenitor cells in patients with emphysema. Proceedings of the American Thoracic Society. 2006;**3**:545-545. DOI: 10.1513/pats.200603-047ms

[31] Borgas D, Chambers E, Newton J, et al. Cigarette smoke disrupted lung endothelial barrier integrity and increased susceptibility to acute lung injury via histone deacetylase 6. American Journal of Respiratory Cell and Molecular Biology. 2016;**54**:683-696. DOI: 10.1165/rcmb.2015-0149OC

[32] U.S. Department of Health and Human Services. How Tobacco Smoke Causes Disease: The Biology and Behavioral Basis of Smoking-Attributable Disease, A Report of the Surgeon General. Rockville, MD: Office of the Surgeon General; 2010. 792 p. ISBN 978-0-16-084078-4. ISBN 10: 0160840783

[33] Patacchini R, Maggi CA. Tachykinins and neurogenic inflammation at visceral level. Neurogenic Inflammation in Health and Disease. 2009;**8**:289-320. DOI: 10.1016/S1567-7443(08)10413-6

[34] Boschetto P, Miotto D, Bononi I, et al. Sputum substance P and neurokinin A are reduced during exacerbations of chronic obstructive pulmonary disease. Pharmacology & Therapeutics. 2005;**18**(3):199-205. DOI: 10.1016/j.pupt.2004.12.006. PMID: 15707854

[35] De Swert KO, Bracke KR, Demoor T, Brusselle GG, Joos GF. Role of the tachykinin NK1 receptor in a murine model of cigarette smoke-induced pulmonary inflammation. Respiratory Research. 2004;**10**(1):37.1-37.3712. DOI: 10.1186/1465-9921-10-37

[36] Almeida TA, Rojo J, Nieto PM, et al. Tachykinins and tachykinin receptors: Structure and activity relationships. Current Medicinal Chemistry. 2004;**11**(15):2045-2081. DOI: 10.2174/0929867043364748

[37] Canning BJ, Spina D. Sensory nerves and airway irritability. Handbook of Experimental Pharmacology. 2009;**194**(194):139-183. DOI: 10.1007/978-3-540-79090-7_5

[38] Joos GF, O'Connor B, Anderson SD, et al. Indirect airway challenges. The European Respiratory Journal. 2003;**21**(6):1050-1068. DOI: 10.1183/09031936.03.00008403

[39] Mapp CE, Miotto D, Braccioni F, et al. The distribution of neurokinin-1 and neurokinin-2 receptors in human central airways. American Journal of Respiratory and Critical Care Medicine. 2000;**161**:207-215. DOI: 10.1007/s11882-001-0081-8

[40] de Swert KO, Joos GF. Extending the understanding of sensory neuropeptides. European Journal of Pharmacology. 2006;**533**(1-3):171-181. DOI: 10.1016/j.ejphar.2005.12.066

[41] D'hulst AI, Vermaelen KY, Brusselle GG, et al. Time course of cigarette smoke-induced pulmonary inflammation in mice. The European Respiratory

Journal. 2005;**26**(2):204-213. DOI: 10.1183/09031936.05.00095204

[42] Kwong KL, Wu ZX, Kashon ML, et al. Chronic smoking enhances tachykinin synthesis and airway responsiveness in guinea pigs. American Journal of Respiratory Cell and Molecular Biology. 2001;**25**(3):299-305. DOI: 10.1165/ajrcmb.25.3.4557

[43] Kharitonov SA, Barnes PJ. Exhaled markers of pulmonary disease. American Journal of Respiratory and Critical Care Medicine. 2001;**163**(7):1693-1722. DOI: 10.1164/ajrccm.163.7.2009041

[44] de Swert KO, Bracke KR, Demoor T, et al. Role of the tachykinin NK1 receptor in a murine model of cigarette smoke-induced pulmonary inflammation. Respiratory Research. 2009;**10**:37. DOI: 10.1186/1465-9921-10-37

[45] Xu J, Xu F. Lin Y Cigarette smoke synergizes lipopolysaccharide-induced interleukin-1β and tumor necrosis factor-α secretion from macrophages via substance P-mediated nuclear factor-κB activation. American Journal of Respiratory Cell and Molecular Biology. 2011;**44**(3):302-308. DOI: 10.1165/rcmb.2009-0288OC. PMID: 20160043

[46] Xu J, Xu F, Wang R, Seagrave J, Lin Y, March TH. Cigarette smoke-induced hypercapnic emphysema in C3H mice is associated with increases of macrophage metalloelastase and substance P in the lungs. Experimental Lung Research. 2007;**33**(5):197-215. DOI: 10.1080/01902140701459514. PMID: 17620183

[47] Schelfhout V, Louis R, Lenz W, et al. The triple neurokinin-receptor antagonist CS-003 inhibits neurokinin A-induced bronchoconstriction in patients with asthma. Pulmonary Pharmacology & Therapeutics. 2006;**19**(6):413-418. DOI: 10.1016/j.pupt.2005.10.007. PMID: 16364669

[48] Tai CF, Baraniuk JN. Upper airway neurogenic mechanisms. Current Opinion in Allergy and Clinical Immunology. 2002;**2**(1):11-19. DOI: 10.1097/00130832-200202000-00003

[49] Groneberg DA, Heppt W, Cryer A, et al. Toxic rhinitis-induced changes of human nasal mucosa innervation. Toxicologic Pathology. 2003;**31**(3):326-331. DOI: 10.1080/01926230390204379

[50] Dinh QT, Klapp BF, Fischer A. Airway sensory nerve and tachykinins in asthma and COPD. Pneumologie. 2006;**60**(2):80-85. DOI: 10.1055/s-2005-915587. PMID: 16463247

[51] Hens G, Raap U, Vanoirbeek J, et al. Selective nasal allergen provocation induces substance P-mediated bronchial hyperresponsiveness. American Journal of Respiratory Cell and Molecular Biology. 2011;**44**(4):517-523. DOI: 10.1165/rcmb.2009-0425OC

[52] Vergnolle N, Cenac N, Altier C, et al. A role for transient receptor potential vanilloid 4 in tonicity-induced neurogenic inflammation. British Journal of Pharmacology. 2010;**159**(5):1161-1173. DOI: 10.1007/s00424-011-1071-x

[53] Zheng H, Liu Y, Huang T, et al. Development and characterization of a rat model of chronic obstructive pulmonary disease (COPD) induced by sidestream cigarette smoke. Toxicology Letters. 2009;**189**(3):225-234. DOI: 10.1016/j.toxlet.2009.06.850. PMID: 19524650

[54] Gilifanov EA, Nevzorova VA, Artyushkin SA, et al. Method for experimental modeling of inflammation in the paranasal sinuses in chronic tobacco smoking in rats. FSBEI HE TSMU Russia. - № 2012121065/14; Pat RU, 2522954, IPC G09B 23/28. - Bull. 2012; No. 20. pp. 1-8

[55] Lee LY, Pisarri TE. Afferent properties and reflex functions

of bronchopulmonary C-fibers. Respiration Physiology. 2001;**125**(1-2):47-65. DOI: 10.1016/S0034-5687(00)00204-8

[56] Ramos-Barbón D, Suzuki M, Taha R, et al. Effect of alpha4-integrin blockade on CD4+ cell-driven late airway responses in the rat. American Journal of Respiratory and Critical Care Medicine. 2001;**163**(1):101-108. PMID: 11208633

[57] Nevzorova VA, Golotina OV, Shekunova OI, et al. Intracardiac and pulmonary hemodynamics and the state of the gas composition of blood with stable angina of stress associated with chronic obstructive pulmonary disease. Cardiovascular Therapy and Prevention. 2011;**10**(8):19-24

[58] Solovyova NI, Ryzhakova OS. Methods for determining the activity of matrix metalloproteinases. Kliniceskaja Laboratornaja Diagnostika. 2010;**16**:17-21

[59] Shoikhet YN, Korenovsky YV, Lepilov AV, et al. The role of matrix metalloproteinases in inflammatory diseases of the lungs. Problems of Clinical Medicine. 2008;**3**:99-101

[60] Atkinson JJ, Senior RM. Matrix metalloproteinase-9 in lung remodeling. American Journal of Respiratory Cell and Molecular Biology. 2003;**28**(1):12-24. DOI: 10.1165/rcmb.2002-0166TR

[61] Ziora D, Dworniczak S, Kozielski J. Induced sputum metalloproteinases and their inhibitors in relation to exhaled nitrogen oxide and sputum nitric oxides and other inflammatory cytokines in patients with chronic obstructive pulmonary disease. Journal of Physiology and Pharmacology. 2008;**59**(6):809-817

[62] Lee WJ, Shin CY, Yoo BK, et al. Induction of matrix metalloproteinase-9 (MMP-9) in lipopolysaccharide-stimulated primary astrocytes is mediated by extracellular signal-regulated protein kinase 1/2 (Erk1/2). Glia. 2003;**41**(1):15-24. PMID: 12465042

[63] Sobolev GM, Sukhikh GT. The family of matrix metalloproteinases: General characteristics and physiological role. Obstetrics and Gynecology. 2007;**1**:5-8

[64] Brodskaya T, Nevzorova V, Zakharchuk N, Repina N. Aortic stiffness and polymorphisms of collagen-1 type 1a gene in COPD patients. Journal of Lung, Pulmonary and Respiratory Research. 2018;**5**(3):81-85. DOI: 10.15406/jlprr.2018.05.00167

Chapter 3

Emphysema

Tomislav M. Jelic

Abstract

Emphysema (Greek word meaning to inflate/to blow) is an increase in the size of airspace distal to the terminal bronchiolus, that is, hyperinflation of the alveoli due to the destruction of the gas-exchanging structures: alveolar walls, alveolar ducts, and respiratory bronchioles with coalescence of airspaces into the abnormal, much larger airspaces. The main consequences are the reduction of alveolar surface for gas exchange and the chronic obstructive pulmonary disease due to the destruction and disappearance of respiratory bronchioles with decreased total small airway diameter sum. Both decreased alveolar surface for gas exchange and chronic obstructive pulmonary disease lead to difficulty in breathing with dyspnea varying from mild to very severe. Two main pathohistologic types of emphysema are centriacinar and panacinar. Centriacinar emphysema involves the central portion of the acinus, and inflation mainly involves respiratory bronchioles and adjacent alveoli, and not all alveoli inside the acinus are involved. Panacinar (panlobular) emphysema is characterized by uniform enlargement and destruction of alveoli throughout the entire acinus. The panacinar emphysema is rare and its most common cause is hereditary alpha-1 antitrypsin deficiency. The centriacinar emphysema is the most frequent emphysema. It is mainly caused by smoking but also by coal dust exposure and advanced age.

Keywords: emphysema, chronic obstructive pulmonary disease, smoking, coal dust, alpha-1 antitrypsin deficiency, oxidative radicals, telomeres

1. Introduction

Emphysema, enlarged airspaces due to destruction of alveolar walls, respiratory bronchioles, and alveolar ducts, is a well-defined disease. However, in the medical practice, it is mainly encountered as an essential component of the chronic obstructive pulmonary disease syndrome. Other components are chronic bronchitis, small airway disease, small airway hyperactivity, and inflammation. Chronic obstructive pulmonary disease presents with cough, sputum production, and exertional dyspnea. In advanced cases, patients are breathless while doing even simple daily activities and may develop resting hypoxemia (blue cyanotic lips and finger nails) that requires continuous application of supplemental oxygen. Chronic obstructive pulmonary disease during its course is complicated by viral, bacterial, and fungal infections, and pneumonias and chronic obstructive pulmonary disease are the fourth leading cause of death in the USA. Urban air pollution and industrial air pollution are contributory factors in the genesis of chronic obstructive pulmonary disease, and with increase in cigarette smoking in developing countries, an estimate is that the chronic obstructive pulmonary disease will rise from the sixth to the third most common cause of death worldwide by the year 2020 [1].

2. Heading

2.1 Morphologic and histologic features of the normal lung

A normal lung consists of airways and alveoli. Airways are tubes (pipes) that conduct air to alveoli where gas exchange occurs. Oxygen (O_2) through alveolar wall enters into red blood cells in the alveolar capillaries and binds to hemoglobin, while carbon dioxide (CO_2) goes in opposite direction being released from hemoglobin, enters alveoli, and is being exhaled.

The trachea beyond the carina undergoes to about 23 generations of dichotomous branching. Airway tubes with diameter of more than 1 mm are called bronchi. With each division the diameter of the bronchus becomes smaller, but the sum of the two diameters exceeds diameter of the parent bronchus meaning that with divisions resistance to air flow becomes smaller. The bronchus consists of the lumen, mucosa, submucosa, muscularis, cartilage, and adventitia that is composed of connective tissue and contains lymphatics (**Figure 1**).

Bronchi are accompanied by branches of the pulmonary artery that have a diameter of similar size to the diameter of the bronchus they follow. The mucosa is mainly lined by columnar respiratory epithelium with cilia. All columnar cells lie on a basement membrane, but since columnar cells differ in their length, nuclei differ in their position regarding basal membrane, and respiratory epithelium appears stratified, but in fact it is pseudostratified. The mucosa also contains small number of mucinous cells that contain apical mucin, small number of basal cells, and rare neuroendocrine cells. Basal cells are precursors of ciliated cells and of mucinous goblet cells. Cilia arise from the apices of the respiratory cells and serve as escalator pushing mucin upstream to the throat and nose. Neuroendocrine cells are scattered singly and form small groups, neuroepithelial bodies near the airway bifurcations. The functional significance of the neuroendocrine cells is largely unknown. Beneath the pseudostratified ciliated mucosa is the submucosa that consists of loose connective tissue harboring bronchial mucous (seromucinous) glands, lymphoid tissue aggregates, and plasma cells. Mucinous glands secrete mucus composed of glycoprotein, proteoglycans, lipids, IgA (secretory) immunoglobulins, lysozyme peroxidase, and other substances to inactivate invading microorganisms, and trap air pollution particles. Cartilage plate and muscle bundles lie beneath the submucosa. The cartilage prevents collapse of the bronchial lumen. There are about 9–12 generations of bronchi. The smallest bronchi are 1 mm in diameter. Bronchi branch into the bronchiole. Bronchioles are less than 1 mm in diameter and they lack cartilage and

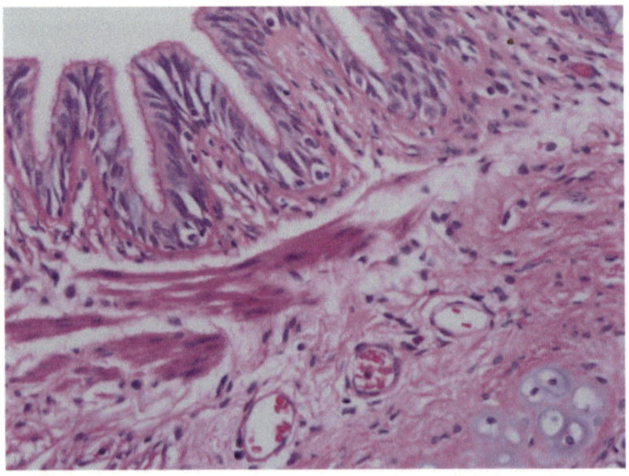

Figure 1.
Portion of the wall of the bronchus with respiratory epithelium with cilia, smooth muscle layer, and cartilage.

exocrine mucinous glands in their walls. The larger bronchioles are called terminal bronchioles and measure on average 0.5–1 mm. Since terminal bronchioles do not contain cartilage, they are also called membranous bronchioles (**Figure 2**).

Terminal bronchioles consist of respiratory mucosa composed of one layer of cuboidal ciliated respiratory cells and occasional Clara cells. Clara cells are non-ciliated columnar epithelial cells with protuberant apical cytoplasm that contains granules of surfactant and protease inhibitors. Clara cells are also precursors of bronchiolar epithelial cells. Goblet cells are generally not present or rare in the mucosa of the terminal bronchioles. Beneath the mucosa of the terminal bronchiolus is a layer of smooth muscle and connective tissue adventitia. Terminal bronchioles branch into the respiratory bronchioles. One side of the airway wall of the respiratory bronchiolus is lined by simple columnar to cuboidal bronchiolar epithelium without cilia. The opposite wall is lined by alveoli, that is, the wall consists of openings of the alveolar sacs. The average diameter of respiratory bronchioles is 0.15–0.2 mm. The respiratory bronchioles branch into about two more generations of respiratory bronchioles. Respiratory bronchioles branch into alveolar ducts, straight tubular spaces bounded entirely by alveoli (**Figure 3**).

In fact all alveoli (alveolar sacs) open into the alveolar ducts. Thus alveoli have incomplete wall and alveolar sacs are outpockets of alveolar ducts. Alveoli that appear lined with alveolar walls on all sides are in fact artifact of cut section. Alveolar ducts are not accompanied by the artery. The acinus is a functional unit of the lungs that consists of terminal bronchiolus with its respiratory bronchioles, alveolar ducts, and alveoli forming tridimensional spherical space with average

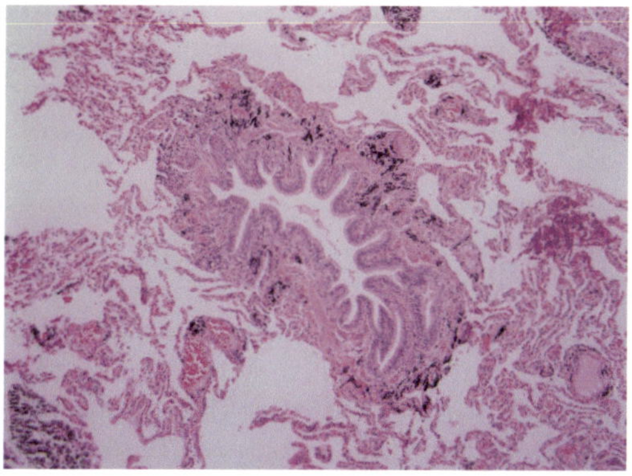

Figure 2.
Terminal bronchiolus, lined by respiratory epithelium, with no cartilage and no exocrine glands.

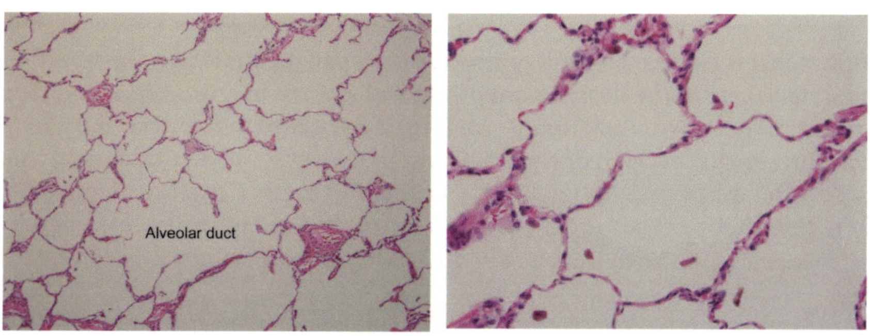

Figure 3.
Alveolar duct and alveoli (original magnification × 100) and alveolar septa with alveoli (original magnification × 400). Courtesy of Dr. Nadia N. Naumova.

diameter of 7.5 mm. There are about three generations of respiratory bronchioles inside the acinus and approximately 25,000 acini in normal adult male lungs with a volume of 5.25 liters [2]. Cluster of three to five terminal bronchioles, that is, acini, form pulmonary lobule. The pulmonary lobule is an anatomic unit, polygonal in shape, and bound by complete or incomplete connective tissue interlobular septa and measures about 1.5–3 cm.

Gas exchange starts in respiratory bronchioles and mainly occurs in alveoli. The alveolar wall (also called alveolar septum) is very thin in order to permit efficient gas exchange (**Figure 3**). It consists only of one layer of epithelial cells called pneumocytes. Pneumocytes type 1 are very thin, flat, large epithelial cells that cover 90% of the alveolar surface and are not capable of mitosis. Pneumocytes type 2 are cuboidal cell with large basal nucleus and prominent nucleolus. Pneumocytes type 2 secrete surfactant, are able to divide and participate in repair, and may become hyperplastic in response to alveolar damage. Pneumocytes type 2 are also precursors of pneumocytes type 1. Pneumocytes lie on the basal membrane that is fused with the basal membrane of the capillary endothelial cell. Thus the alveolar wall (septum) consists only of capillary sandwiched between the two layers of pneumocytes from two adjacent alveoli (**Figure 3**). An occasional myofibroblast may be present in the alveolar wall as well as rare scattered small lymphocytes, rare mesenchymal cells, and rare macrophages. Hematoxylin and eosin-stained sections of the normal lung on high magnification show delicate alveolar walls (septa) containing inconspicuous capillaries, occasional cuboidal cells of pneumocytes type 2, and nuclei of pneumocytes type 1, endothelial cell nuclei, and nuclei of rare scattered lymphocytes, mesenchymal cells, and macrophages. The cytoplasm of pneumocytes type 1 is too thin to be visible without special immunoperoxidase stains. Alveolar macrophages egress from capillaries, are increased in number in chronic inflammatory settings, and are involved in phagocytosis of foreign material as well in the inflammatory and immune responses.

The interstitium provides the connective tissue framework of the lungs and is composed of collagen fibers, elastic fibers, mesenchymal cells, and few inflammatory cells. In normal lungs the interstitium is generally inconspicuous and can be recognized only along bronchovascular bundles, around veins, and where it forms interlobular septa. In the children up to 4 years of age, the interstitium is more apparent and presents as thickening of the alveolar walls [3]. The term “small airways” includes airways with diameter of 2 mm and smaller and thus includes small bronchi, terminal bronchioles, and respiratory bronchioles.

2.2 Morphologic and histologic features of emphysema

Emphysema is permanent enlargement of airspaces distal to the terminal bronchiole (acinus) due to the destruction of the walls of the alveoli, alveolar ducts, and the respiratory bronchioles. Grossly, the lung is hyperinflated and spongy.

According to the location of the hyperinflated alveoli inside the acinus, there are four types of emphysema: centriacinar (centrilobular, proximal), panacinar (panlobular), distal acinar (paraseptal), and irregular (associated with scar). Each of the emphysema type has characteristic microscopic morphology and characteristic etiology.

The most frequent is centriacinar emphysema which comprises more than 95% of all emphysemas. **Centriacinar emphysema** involves proximal respiratory bronchiolus and adjacent alveoli, which is in the center of the acinus, hence the name centriacinar emphysema (**Figure 4**).

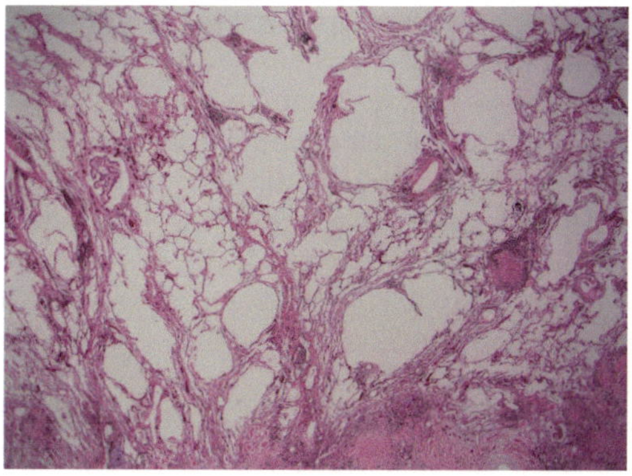

Figure 4.
Centriacinar emphysema caused by coal mine dust. Some alveoli are normal, some emphysematous. Hematoxylin and eosin stain, original magnification 20×.

Inhaled cigarette smoke or mineral dust, most frequently coal mine dust, reach respiratory bronchioles. There are no cilia in the respiratory bronchioles; cigarette smoke particles and coal dust particles (silica particles in the coal dust are the most toxic ones) stick there and initiate processes of inflammation and destruction. The first damaged structure is thus respiratory bronchiolus with its dilatation or disappearance. In the beginning, alveolar ducts and alveoli are spared. Soon their destruction and coalescence into the larger air space follows. In the acinus, which contains several (about 14) respiratory bronchioles, some bronchioles and alveoli are damaged, enlarged, and emphysematous, and some are not damaged and are normal in size. Thus characteristic microscopic feature with low power magnification of centroacinar emphysema is that some alveoli are normal and some emphysematous (**Figures 4** and 5).

Cigarette smoke produces similar damage, and in fact the most frequent cause of centriacinar emphysema is cigarette smoking. Centriacinar emphysema predominantly involves the upper and posterior portions of the lungs and upper parts of the individual lobes. In severe emphysema, emphysematous spaces may coalesce and form bullae which may reach several centimeters in diameters. By definition bulla is at least 1 cm in diameter. Bullae are usually located in the lung apices and subpleurally but can occur anywhere in the emphysematous lungs.

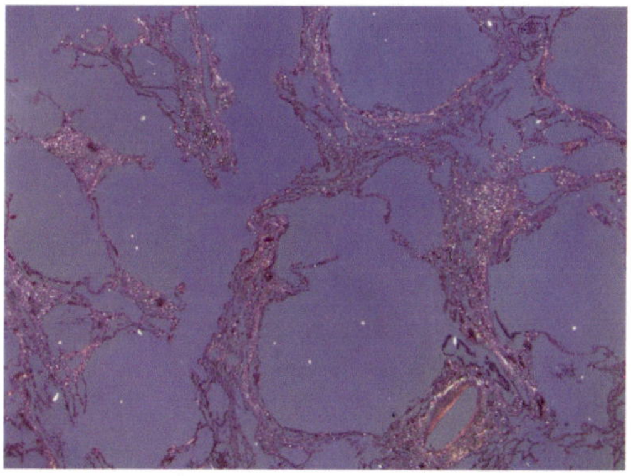

Figure 5.
Centriacinar emphysema and interstitial fibrosis caused by birefringent silica/silicate particles from coal mine dust. This is the same area as in **Figure 4***, but with original magnification × 400 and photographed under polarized light to highlight birefringent silica/silicate particles; small white dots in the interstitium and silvery collagen fibers of interstitial (septal alveolar) fibrosis.*

Panacinar emphysema (panlobular emphysema) comprises 1% of emphysemas. It involves the entire acinus, that is, all alveoli in the acinus are about equally dilated, and all acini in the lobule are involved by panacinar (panlobular) emphysema (**Figure 6**). In centriacinar emphysema, some alveoli are enlarged and some are normal.

Panacinar emphysema is associated with alpha-1-antitrypsin deficiency, an autosomal codominant genetic disorder. Since defect is present in the gene (chromosome 14, segment q32.1), every cell, in which this gene is active and its product anti-protease alpha-1 antitrypsin enzyme pertinent, is affected. Thus all respiratory bronchioles, alveolar ducts, and alveoli are affected and about equally damaged and equally hyperinflated. The lungs are diffusely affected by panacinar emphysema, and histologically there is diffuse enlargement of the alveoli affecting the entire acinus. Normal level of alpha-1 antitrypsin in the serum is 20–48 μM/L. P atients with emphysema have concentration of serum alpha-1 antitrypsin 2.5–7 μM/L, and they are homozygous for PI*ZZ allele (PI* denotes protein inhibitor gene). There are more than 90 different alleles of PI* gene, and some variants cause a change in conformation of the alpha-1-antitrypsin molecule leading to polymerization and retention of misshaped protein in hepatocytes (major site of synthesis of alpha-1 antitrypsin) that might lead in children as well in adults to cirrhosis of the liver. If there is absence of protein inhibitor gene, serum level of alpha-1 antitrypsin is zero. Panacinar emphysema might also occur in intravenous drug abusers and then is accompanied with talc granulomas and interstitial fibrosis [3, 4]. Birefringent particles of talk could be seen under polarized light in the granulomas and in the fibrotic interstitium (**Figure 7**).

Distal acinar emphysema (paraseptal emphysema) involves distal part of the acinus including alveolar ducts and alveoli. It is rare. Distal acinar emphysema is most often present in the upper lobes beneath the pleura and along septa between lobules and also is called paraseptal, subpleural, or localized emphysema. The pathogenesis of distal acinar emphysema is unknown. Distal acinar emphysema produces apical bullae which may cause spontaneous pneumothorax in young adults.

Irregular emphysema is airspace enlargement due to lung destruction associated with scarring, also termed scar emphysema, paracicatrical emphysema, and perifocal emphysema. Foci of irregular emphysema are asymptomatic and clinically insignificant. The National Heart, Lung, and Blood Institute does not regard irregular emphysema as a form of emphysema but as "airspace enlargement with fibrosis" [5].

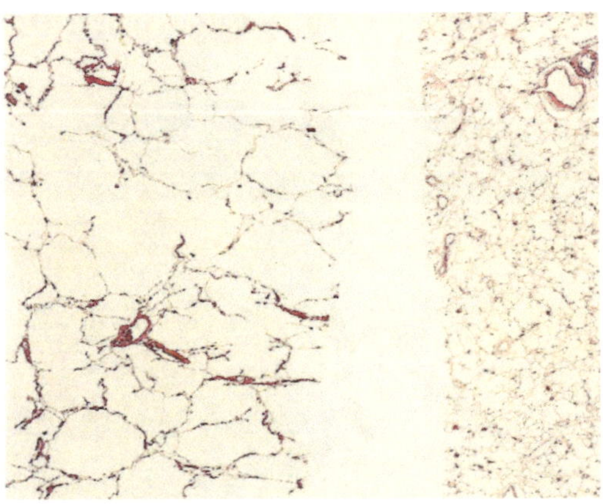

Figure 6.
Panacinar emphysema (left) and normal lung (right). In panacinar emphysema, all alveoli are enlarged. Figure 6, is reproduced with permission from the American Registry of Pathology from the Atlas of Nontumor Pathology Series; Non-Neoplastic Disorders of the Lower Respiratory Tract by William D. Travis et al published by the American Registry of Pathology and the Armed Forces Institute of Pathology Washington DC, USA, Copyright© 2002.

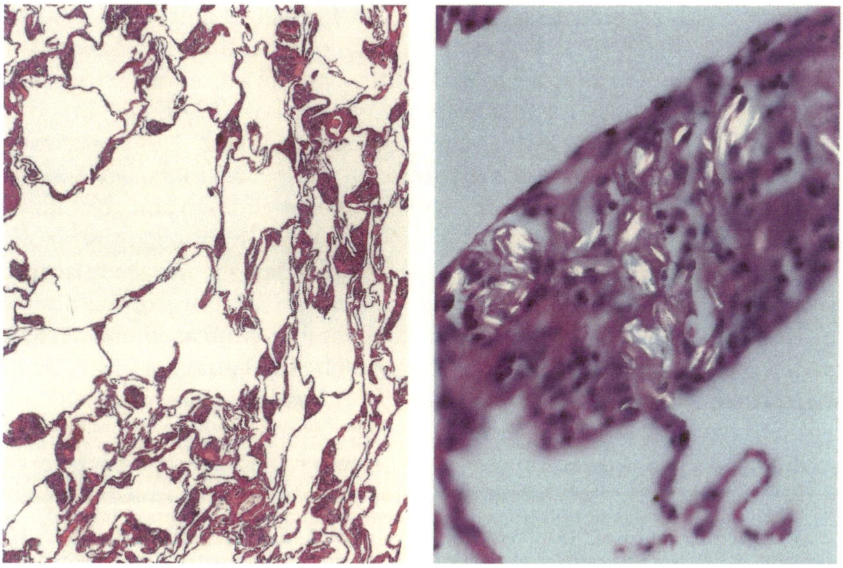

Figure 7.
Panacinar emphysema caused by drug abuse. Mild interstitial fibrosis is present as well as birefringent deposits of talc in the interstitium. Figure 7 is reproduced with permission from the American Registry of Pathology from the Atlas of Nontumor Pathology Series; Non-Neoplastic Disorders of the Lower Respiratory Tract by William D. Travis et al published by the American Registry of Pathology and the Armed Forces Institute of Pathology Washington DC, USA, Copyright© 2002.

The pathogenesis of centriacinar and panacinar emphysema is conceptually similar and based on proteinase-antiproteinase imbalance, that is, inequity between enzymes that degrade the extracellular matrix and proteins that oppose this proteolytic activity [6]. The first clue appeared in 1963 when Laurell and Eriksson identified patients with alpha-1 antitrypsin (more appropriate name is alpha-1 antiproteinase) deficiency on serum electrophoresis who had severe emphysema of early onset and in 1964 when Gross and coworkers demonstrated that proteolytic enzyme papain can produce emphysema in rats [7, 8]. Alpha-1 antitrypsin is a proteinase inhibitor that inhibits proteolytic enzymes, primarily neutrophil elastase. Elastase is an enzyme that destroys elastin fibers, and if it is not adequately inhibited by alpha-1 antitrypsin, destruction of acinar tissue follows leading to emphysema. Imbalance between other proteolytic enzymes (metalloproteinases including interstitial collagenase-1, interstitial collagenase-3, metalloelastase, matrilysin, gelatinase A and gelatinase B, cathepsins) and their inhibitors (tissue inhibitors of matrix metalloproteinases, elafin, epithelium-derived secretory leukoprotease inhibitor) also contributes to emphysema and chronic obstructive pulmonary disease [3, 6].

Cigarette smoking is the most frequent cause of emphysema and accounts to 80–90% of chronic obstructive pulmonary disease cases in the USA [9]. Cigarette smoke and coal mine dust cause emphysema by a similar pathophysiologic pathway. Inhaled cigarette smoke as well as coal mining dust particles travel by airflow to respiratory bronchioles and alveoli where they interfere with epithelial cells, alveolar macrophages, and neutrophils. Cigarette smoke contains per puff an estimated 10^{15}–10^{17} oxidants/free radicals and about 4700 different chemical compounds, including reactive aldehydes and quinones [10, 11]. Toxic oxidant compounds in cigarette smoke induce DNA damage and peroxidation of lipids, harm proteins, fold proteins, and cause them to aggregate in the cytoplasm of the respiratory cells and alveolar cells [12]. Alveolar epithelial cells and macrophages damaged by cigarette smoke release cytokines which invite inside alveoli inflammatory cells mainly macrophages but also T cells (T8 more than T4) and small number of neutrophils. Characteristic histologic findings in cigarette smokers are tobacco-associated respiratory bronchiolitis with the presence of macrophages containing smoker granules (yellow-brown) inside alveoli (**Figure 8**). Macrophages and neutrophils activated by cigarette smoke or silica (quartz) [13] particles in coal mine dust release abovementioned proteolytic enzymes that destroy collagen and elastic alveolar tissue causing connective tissue breakdown and alveolar tissue destruction, that is, emphysema [14]. Oxidative radicals in the cigarette smoke as well as quartz-generated hydrogen peroxide not only damage intracellular proteins but also inactivate alpha-1 antitrypsin by oxidizing the SH group of methionine to methionine sulfoxide [14]. Other proteins, for example, proteasome with caspase-like activity, are also impaired by this oxidation. The final effect of cigarette smoke and inhalation of coal mine dust is unopposed (or insufficiently inhibited) action of proteolytic enzymes that destroy lung parenchyma and cause emphysema.

Macrophages also produce transforming growth factor-beta, platelet-derived growth factor, and tumor necrosis-alpha, which all stimulate fibroblast growth, collagen production and repair with associated fibrosis [15]. Repair may not be perfect and interstitial fibrosis may occur. Bronchioles and small bronchi can be involved by fibrosis and contribute to the chronic obstructive pulmonary disease. Tobacco-caused respiratory bronchiolitis-associated interstitial lung disease with fibrosis (**Figure 9**) is now a plausible and established term [16, 17].

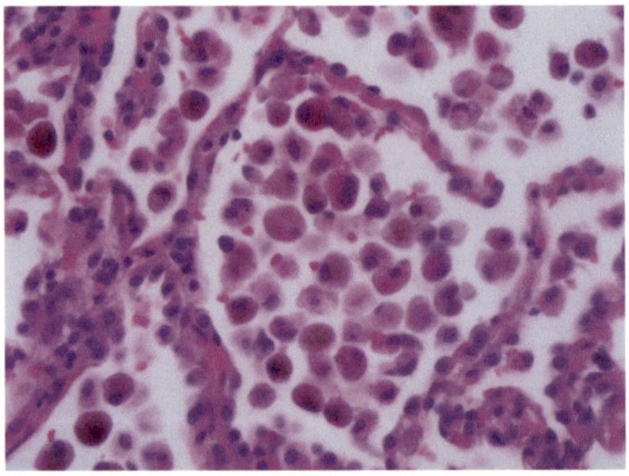

Figure 8.
Tobacco-associated respiratory bronchiolitis. Macrophages with smoker granules inside alveoli. Hematoxylin and eosin stain, original magnification 400×.

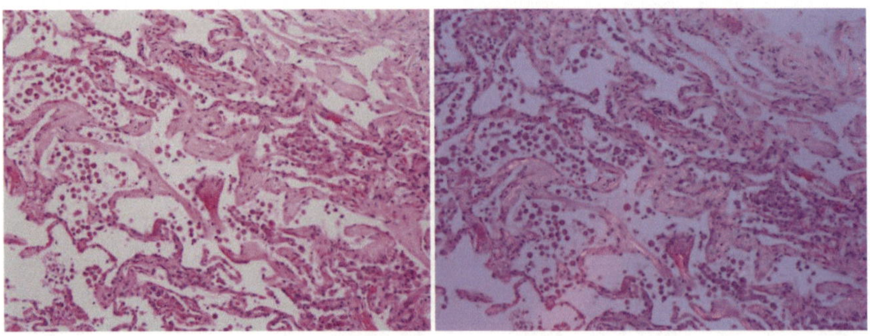

Figure 9.
Tobacco-associated respiratory bronchiolitis with interstitial fibrosis. Hematoxylin and eosin stain, original magnification 200×. Right, same picture under polarized light to demonstrate collagen (silvery shine) fibers in thickened fibrotic alveolar septa.

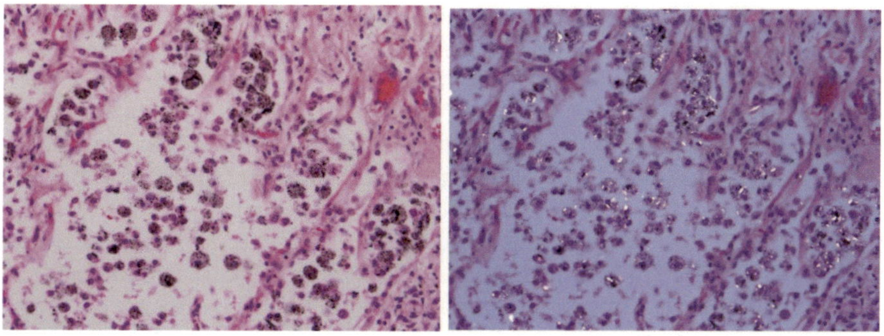

Figure 10.
Initial event in development of emphysema and interstitial fibrosis in coal miners is appearance of macrophages laden with silica and silicate particles and anthracotic pigment inside alveoli. Hematoxylin and eosin stain, original magnification 400×. Right side, same picture under polarized light to demonstrate birefringent silica and silicate particles in the cytoplasm of macrophages. Very small and faint white dots are silica particles, and small bright dots are silicate particles.

It is obvious that tobacco-associated emphysema and tobacco-associated interstitial fibrosis are related and that the first step in their genesis is accumulation of macrophages with smoker granules in the alveoli. The similar process can be elicited by silica and silicates from coal mine dust. The first sign of exposure to coal mine dust is accumulation of silica/silicate particles and anthracotic pigment in the alveolar macrophages (**Figure 10**) [18].

In coal miners with complicated coal worker's pneumoconiosis, the role of smoking in causing fibrosis is insignificant in comparison with that of silica/silicate particles from coal mine dust [18]. Since smoking and coal mine dust simultaneously may cause pulmonary fibrosis and emphysema by destruction of lung tissue and healing by fibrosis, it is plausible that in some patients emphysema is dominant, in others interstitial fibrosis, and in some others combined pulmonary fibrosis and emphysema syndrome (**Figure 11**) may occur [18, 19].

Alpha-1 antitrypsin deficiency is not the only one known genetic cause of emphysema. Telomere length is also associated with emphysema [20]. Both tips (ends) of the chromosomes are capped (protected) by telomeres composed of tandemly repeated DNA sequences. Telomeres are highly conserved and practically identical from protozoa to vertebrates. In humans, the TTAGGG repeat region is 10–15 kilobytes long. With each mitosis terminal nucleotides at the tail of telomeres are lost, and telomeres become shorter with each cell division. When telomere becomes critically short, the cell cannot

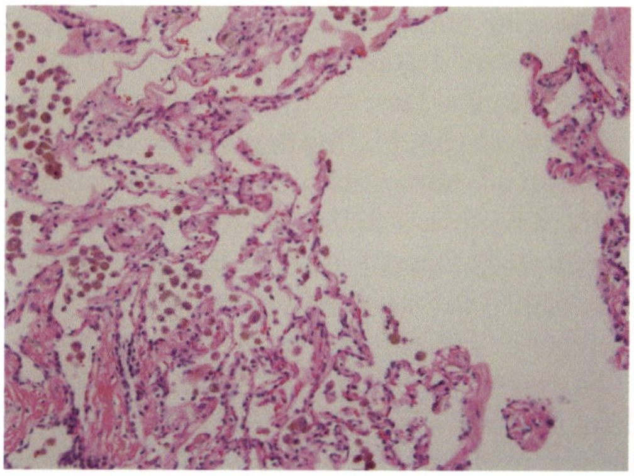

Figure 11.
Tobacco caused emphysema and tobacco caused respiratory bronchiolitis-associated interstitial lung disease with fibrosis, called combined pulmonary fibrosis and emphysema syndrome. Courtesy of Dr. Nadia N. Naumova.

divide anymore and thus becomes an old cell that will finally end up in apoptosis. Telomerase is an enzyme that synthesizes telomeres. Mutations in telomerase gene and telomere genes cause short telomere length for cell age and disease spectrum called short telomere syndrome/accelerated aging syndrome. The main presentation (90%) of short telomere syndromes are idiopathic pulmonary (interstitial) fibrosis and emphysema. They may be associated with other features of premature aging including early graying, osteoporosis, liver disease, predisposition to bone marrow failure, infertility, as well as myelodysplastic syndrome and acute myeloid leukemia [21]. Reduced telomere length may be identified in 25% of patients with sporadic idiopathic pulmonary fibrosis and half of those cases with family aggregation [22]. Telomerase deficiency and telomere shortening are responsible for only 1% of all emphysemas but are conceptually important as a link between interstitial fibrosis, emphysema, combined emphysema and interstitial fibrosis, and effect of environment on phenotypic presentation of genetic defect [21]. Pathogenic mechanism is premature senescence of alveolar epithelial stem cells, their apoptosis, disappearance of alveoli (emphysema), and abnormal repair with excessive interstitial fibrosis. The same genetic change, germline deletion in the Box H domain of the RNA telomerase, can cause in the father idiopathic pulmonary fibrosis, in one daughter emphysema, and in the other daughter combined pulmonary fibrosis and emphysema syndrome [20]. Interaction between the gene and environment determines lung disease. Never-smokers develop pulmonary interstitial fibrosis, while smokers develop an early onset emphysema alone or combined emphysema and pulmonary interstitial fibrosis [20, 21]. Cigarette smoke causes additive DNA damage to telomere function, and genetic defect in this setting expresses as emphysema [20].

In short, the main causes of emphysema and interstitial fibrosis are cigarette smoking and in coal miners silica and silicate particles from coal dust. Hereditary emphysemas caused by alpha-1 antitrypsin deficiency and short telomere length are epidemiologically insignificant but can help to elucidate pathogenesis of emphysema and interstitial fibrosis. Not all smokers develop emphysema and chronic obstructive pulmonary disease. Only 10–20% of the smokers develop chronic obstructive pulmonary disease pointing at an additional risk factor such as genetic susceptibility reflected in polymorphisms in genes coding for various antiproteases, a disintegrin, and metalloproteinase 33 or antioxidant superoxide dismutase and proinflammatory mediators including tumor necrosis factor-alpha [10] and possibly genes associated with telomeres. Combined pulmonary fibrosis and emphysema are also in the vast majority of cases caused by cigarette smoking or in coal miners by coal dust, and the above mentioned genetic factors might contribute to a now unknown degree of susceptibility.

Patients with emphysema only are extremely rare, and in practice emphysema is component of the chronic obstructive pulmonary disease which affects about 24 million people in the USA. Chronic bronchitis is chronic mucous hypersecretion syndrome and is clinically defined as productive cough for at least 3 months in 2 successive years. Its pathohistological features (**Figure 12**) include enlargement of the mucus-secreting glands in the bronchial wall, goblet cell metaplasia of the respiratory epithelium, infiltration of the bronchial mucosa with lymphocytes, squamous metaplasia and dysplasia in the bronchial epithelium, increased bronchial smooth muscle, as well as mucous plugging, inflammation, and fibrosis of the bronchioles.

Chronic bronchitis becomes chronic obstructive bronchitis when airflow obstruction occurs. It can be detected by spirometry or expiratory wheezing can be heard by auscultation. Bronchial airways are being compressed during expiration, and expiration is in chronic obstructive bronchitis difficult and prolonged. Auscultation reveals diminished breath sounds, prolonged expiratory phase, and expiratory wheezing. The main airflow obstruction occurs in small airways, with diameter less than 2 mm. Obstruction is caused by mucosal thickening, due to lymphocytic infiltration, fibrosis, edema, mucous plugging, and smooth muscle hypertrophy. **Figure 13** demonstrates

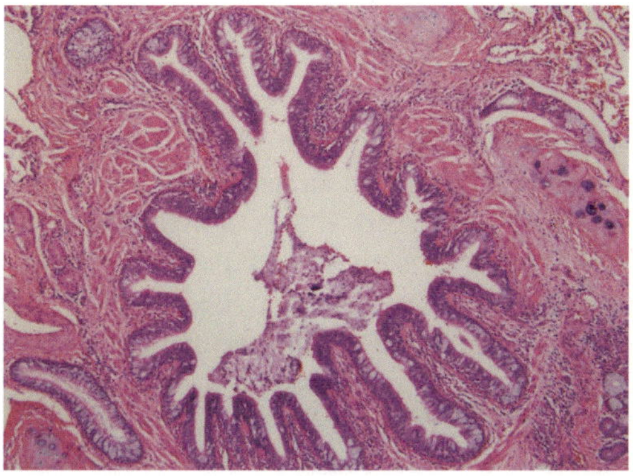

Figure 12.
Chronic bronchitis presenting with mucus in the lumen of the bronchus, partial goblet cell metaplasia of the respiratory epithelium, predominance of the mucinous cells in the bronchial exocrine gland, infiltration the bronchial wall by small lymphocytes and plasma cells, hypertrophy of the muscle layer, and peribronchial fibrosis.

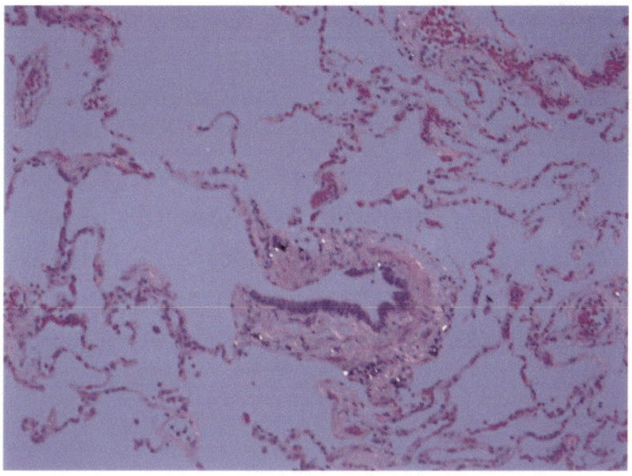

Figure 13.
The wall of the terminal bronchiolus is thickened by fibrosis and smooth muscle hypertrophy and this is one of the essential pathologic bases for obstructive pulmonary disease. Birefringent silica and silicate particles are etiological factor. Hematoxylin and eosin stain, original magnification 200×, polarized light.

thickening of the wall of the terminal bronchiolus by fibrous tissue and smooth muscle hypertrophy caused by birefringent silica/silicate particles from coal mine dust.

Clara cells that secrete surfactant are replaced by goblet cells, and decrease of surfactant increases surface tension at the air-tissue interface, and small bronchi and bronchiole are prone to collapse. Emphysema also contributes to airflow obstruction. Destruction and disappearance of respiratory bronchiole and alveolar ducts decrease total airway diameter. Destruction of acinar tissue with disappearance of elastic fibers decreases lung recoil and decreases expiratory air force. The net effect of chronic obstructive pulmonary disease is difficulty in breathing, prolonged expiration with expiratory wheezing, air trapping in the lungs with hyperinflation of lungs, increased residual volume, decreased vital capacity, and dyspnea.

Three cardinal features of chronic obstructive pulmonary disease are cough, sputum production, and exertional dyspnea. Dyspnea during physical activity may start insidiously, and patients complain of difficult breathing, gasping and air hunger, heaviness in chest in the beginning only during rather heavy physical work and later during light daily physical activity. Patients with chronic obstructive pulmonary disease poorly tolerate physical activity with arms but tolerate better physical work like pushing shopping cart when arms are fixed and enable the use of accessory respiratory muscles [1]. Acute exacerbations of chronic obstructive pulmonary disease are prominent feature of its natural history and are characterized by cough, increase in amount and character (color) of sputum, and dyspnea and may or may not be accompanied with fever, myalgia, and sore throat. The health-related quality of life of patients with chronic obstructive pulmonary disease better correlates (inverse correlation) with frequency of acute exacerbations than with the degree of airflow obstruction (Reilly-Harrison). Patients with advanced emphysema due to hyperinflation of lungs have barrel chest with poor diaphragmatic excursion as assessed by percussion and dramatic decrease in breath sounds and are sitting in the characteristic tripod position with stretched fixed arms to enable the use of accessory respiratory muscles including sternocleidomastoid, scalene, and intercostal ones [1]. Patients with predominant emphysema are called "pink puffers" because they breathe through pursed lips with the help of accessory respiratory muscles. When small airway obstruction ensues, patients become hypoxic and cyanotic in the lips and nail beds, and when fluid retains due to right heart decompensation, they become "blue bloaters." However the majority of chronic obstructive pulmonary disease patients have some signs of both, "pink puffers" and "blue bloaters." Advanced chronic obstructive lung disease is accompanied by systemic wasting due to high energy expenditure for increased work of breathing muscles including accessory breathing muscles and elevated levels of inflammatory cytokines including tumor necrosis factor-alpha. Such patients have a significant weight loss and diffuse loss of subcutaneous fatty tissue. Some patients with advanced chronic obstructive pulmonary disease have paradoxical inward movement of the lower rib cage (Hoover sign) due to diaphragmatic contraction in a setting of permanently hyperinflated lungs [1]. Advanced chronic obstructive pulmonary disease, especially during acute exacerbation, can be accompanied by right heart failure. Signs include right ventricular heave, third heart sound, distended jugular veins, congested liver, ascites, and edema of legs.

2.3 Radiologic findings

Cardinal features of emphysema, hyperinflation of the lungs, and lung tissue destruction can be visualized by radiologic means. On the chest roentgenogram hyperinflation presents with increased lucency, increased retrosternal air space, depression and flattening of the diaphragm. Lung destruction presents in focal lucencies and areas of decreased vascularity. Mild emphysema is usually missed by standard chest X-rays.

High-resolution computerized tomography is superior to the chest X-ray in detecting emphysema. High-resolution computerized tomography can visualize focal areas of decreased attenuation sharply circumscribed without visible walls and with small centrilobular vessel in the areas of emphysema [3]. Several studies showed good correlation between the degree of pathologic findings and high-resolution computerized tomography findings [23]. However, mild focal areas might not be detected, and high-resolution computerized tomography cannot be used to rule out emphysema [24].

2.4 Tests of pulmonary function

Spirometry and pulse oximetry are basic simple pulmonary function tests that can be performed in the ambulatory settings. The patient exhales in the spirometry instrument as completely as possible, then forcibly inhales as much as possible, and then forcibly exhales as much as possible. Forced vital capacity is the maximum amount of air forcibly expired after maximum inspiration. Residual volume is amount of air retained in the lungs after maximal and forceful exhalation, and it can be calculated after using gas dilution technique or body-box plethysmography. In the emphysema due to the destruction of respiratory bronchioles, spirometry will demonstrate obstructive pattern. Forced expiratory volume in 1 second will be decreased. Alveolar destruction in emphysema decreases amount of lung parenchyma, and thus forced vital capacity will decrease. Essentially emphysema is a mixed lung disorder, both obstructive and restrictive.

Transcutaneous pulse oximetry estimates oxygen (O_2) saturation of capillary blood using instrument in shape of clip positioned on a finger. Estimation is accurate and correlates to 5% of measured atrial O_2 saturation obtained by invasive procedure.

2.5 Therapy

Centriacinar emphysema is a progressive disabling disease for which there are no good therapeutic options. Large bullae that compress functional lung tissue can be surgically removed. Patients with severe, predominantly upper lung emphysema, and low baseline exercise capacity may benefit from lung volume reduction by resection, including bronchoscopic lung volume reduction, of non-functioning emphysematous areas. Dyspnea decreases because of reduced hyperinflation and residual volume and because forced expiration volume in the first second is increased [25]. Exercise tolerance and 2-year mortality rate are improved supposedly to decreased residual lung volume, enhanced lung recoil, and improved diaphragmatic function. Long-term effects of the lung volume reduction surgery are unknown. Improvement after lung transplantation is better than after the lung volume reduction surgery. Candidates for lung transplantation are younger than 60 years, with an FEV_1 less than 25% predicted or pulmonary artery hypertension. The 5-year survival after transplantation for emphysema is 45–60%. Lifelong immunosuppression brings risk of opportunistic infections.

Conflicts of interest

None declared.

Author details

Tomislav M. Jelic
Department of Pathology and Laboratory Medicine, Charleston Area Medical Center, Charleston, West Virginia, USA

*Address all correspondence to: tomsilav.jelic@camc.org

References

[1] Reilly J, Silverman E, Shapiro S. Chronic obstructive pulmonary disease. In: Kasper D, Fauci A, Longo D, Braunwald E, Hauser S, Jameson LJ, editors. Harrison's Principles of Internal Medicine. 16th ed. New York: McGraw-Hill; 2005. pp. 1547-1554

[2] Sorokin SP. The respiratory system. In: Weiss L, editor. Cell and Tissue Biology. 6th ed. Baltimore: Urban & Schwarzenberg; 1988. pp. 753-814

[3] Travis W, Colby T, Koss M, de Christenson R, Muller N, King T Jr. Non-Neoplastic Disorders of the Lower Respiratory Tract. Atlas of Nontumor Pathology. AFIP, ARP. pp. 435-471

[4] Schmidt RA, Glenny RW, Godwin JD, Hampson NB, Cantino ME, Reichenbach DD. Panlobular emphysema in young intravenous Ritalin abusers. The American Review of Respiratory Disease. 1991;**143**:649-646

[5] Snider GL, Kleinerman J, Thurlbeck WM, Bengali ZH. The definition of emphysema. Report of a National Heart , Lung, and Blood Institute, Division of Lung Diseases workshop. The American Review of Respiratory Disease. 1985;**132**:182-185

[6] Pardo A, Selman M. Proteinase-antiproteinase imbalance in the pathogenesis of Emphysema: The role of metalloproteinases in lung damage. Histology and Histopathology. 1999;**14**:227-233

[7] Laurell CB, Eriksson S. The electrophoretical alpha1-globulin pattern of serum alpha1-antitrypsin deficiency. Scandinavian Journal of Clinical and Laboratory Investigation. 1963;**15**:132-140

[8] Gross P, Pfitzer EA, Tolker E, Babyok MA, Kaschak M. Experimental emphysema, its production with papain in normal and silicotic rats. Archives of Environmental Health. 1965;**11**:50-58

[9] Sethi S, Rochesert CL. Smoking and chronic obstructive pulmonary disease. Clinics in Chest Medicine. 2000;**21**:67-86

[10] Hongwei Y, Rahman I. Current concepts on oxidative/carbonyl stress, inflammation and epigenetics in pathogenesis of chronic obstructive pulmonary disease. Toxicology and Applied Pharmacology. 2011;**254**(2):72-85

[11] Church DF, Pryor WA. Free-radical chemistry of cigarette smoke and its toxicological implications. Environmental Health Perspectives. 1985;**64**:111-126

[12] Tran I, Ji C, Ni I, Min T, Tang D, Vij N. Role of cigarette smoke-induced aggresome formation in chronic obstructive pulmonary disease-emphysema pathogenesis. American Journal of Respiratory Cell and Molecular Biology. 2015;**53**(2):159-173

[13] Cohen RA, Petsonk EL, Rose C, et al. Lung pathology in U.S. coal workers with rapidly progressive pneumoconiosis implicates silica and silicates. American Journal of Respiratory and Critical Care Medicine. 1964;(6):673-680

[14] Churg A, Zay K, Li K. Mechanisms of mineral dust-induced emphysema. Environmental Health Perspectives. 1997;**105**(Suppl 5):1215-1218

[15] Schns RP, Borm PJ. Mechanisms and mediators in coal dust induced toxicity: a review. The Annals of Occupational Hygiene. 1999;**43**(1):7-33

[16] Vassalllo R, Ryu JH. Tobacco smoke-related diffuse lung diseases. Seminars in Respiratory and Critical Care Medicine. 2008;**29**(6):643-650

[17] Yousem SA. Respiratory bronchiolitis-associated interstitial lung disease with fibrosis is a lesion distinct from fibrotic nonspecific interstitial pneumonia: a proposal. Modern Pathology. 2006;(11):1474-1479

[18] Jelic TM, Estalilla OC, Sawyer-Kaplan PR, Plata MJ, Powers JT, Emmett M, et al. Coal mine dust desquamative chronic interstitial pneumonia: A precursor of dust-related diffuse fibrosis and of emphysema. International Journal of Occupational and Environmental Medicine. 2017;**8**(3):153-165

[19] Jankowich MD, Rounds SI. Combined pulmonary fibrosis and emphysema syndrome: a review. Chest. 2012;**141**:222-231

[20] Alder JK, Guo N, Parry EM, Anderson CJ, Gorgy AI, Walshg MF, et al. Telomere length is a determinant of emphysema susceptibility. American Journal of Respiratory and Critical Care Medicine. 2011;**184**:904-912

[21] Stanley SE, Merck SJ, Armanios M. Telomerase and genetics of emphysema susceptibility. Implications for pathogenesis paradigms and patient care. Annals of the American Thoracic Society. 2016;**13**(Suppl 5):S447-S451

[22] Molina-Molina M, Borie R. Clinical implications of telomere dysfunction in lung fibrosis. Current Opinion in Pulmonary Medicine. 2018;**24**(5):440-444

[23] Hruban RH, Meziane MA, Zerhouni EA, et al. High resolution computerized tomography of inflation-fixed lungs. Pathologic-radiologic correlation of centrilobular emphysema. The American Review of Respiratory Disease. 1987;**136**:935-940

[24] Miller RR, Muller NL, Vedal S, Morrison NJ, Staples CA. Limitations of computed tomography in the assessment of emphysema. The American Review of Respiratory Disease. 1989;**139**:980-983

[25] Gulsen A. Bronchoscopic lung volume reduction: A 2018 review and update. Turkish Thoracic Journal. 2018;**19**(3):141-149

Chapter 4

COPD Pharmacological Management Update

Stefan-Marian Frent

Abstract

Chronic obstructive pulmonary disease (COPD) is a significant cause of morbidity and mortality worldwide. Although it is considered both preventable and treatable, COPD still represents an important public health challenge. The classes of pharmacological agents widely used for the maintenance treatment are bronchodilators (SABA, SAMA, LABA, LAMA) and inhaled corticosteroids (ICS). While it is largely accepted that inhaled bronchodilators, which are effective and well tolerated in patients with stable disease, are the cornerstone of the pharmacological management of COPD, there is an ongoing debate regarding the role of inhaled corticosteroids. This is also reflected in the last versions of the GOLD recommendations, which suffered dramatic changes in the recent years. The trend for personalized medicine led to the search for biomarkers which could guide the therapeutic decisions. Recent studies demonstrated that blood eosinophils can reasonably predict the ICS relative efficacy in preventing COPD exacerbations and thus could inform the disease management.

Keywords: COPD, lung function, exacerbation, bronchodilators, corticosteroids, biomarkers, eosinophils

1. Introduction

Chronic Obstructive Pulmonary Disease (COPD) is a common condition, usually affecting people of >40 years of age significantly exposed to noxious particles or gases [1]. Although considered both preventable and treatable [1], COPD remains a leading cause of morbidity and mortality [2, 3], affecting an estimated 384 million people worldwide [4]. The COPD prevalence is projected to increase in the coming decades [5], as well as its position among the leading causes of mortality [4].

Active or passive cigarette smoking is the most commonly encountered risk factor for COPD across the world [1]; however other factors may play a role in the disease pathogenesis, such as genetic factors [6, 7], exposure to indoor and outdoor air pollutants [8–11], exposure to occupational dusts, chemical agents or fumes [12], infections (HIV, tuberculosis) [13, 14], and socioeconomic status [15].

The normal lung response to the inhalation of noxious factors is an inflammatory reaction of the airways. In patients who develop COPD, the excessive inflammatory response is further enhanced by the oxidative stress and an imbalance of the protease-antiprotease system, leading to the destruction of the lung parenchyma and disruption of normal repair and defense mechanisms. Emphysema and small airway fibrosis are the consequences of these processes, which translate into gas trapping and chronic airflow limitation [1].

By definition, COPD is a chronic condition, and the major symptoms exhibited by the patients suffering from this disease, dyspnea, cough, and sputum production, are usually persistent and/or progressive and have a considerable negative effect on the patient's quality of life. The Global Burden of Disease Study highlighted that COPD is a major contributor to disability and mortality around the world, by ranking COPD as the fifth leading cause of disability-adjusted life years (DALYs) lost in 2013 [16].

The natural course of the disease is grafted by acute episodes of worsening of symptoms triggered by infectious agents, air pollution, and other factors. These events are referred to as "exacerbations" and usually require a change in medication and/or hospitalization. Exacerbations are associated with accelerated lung function decline, reduced quality of life, and increased mortality [17] and, not surprisingly, have been surnamed as "chest attacks" or "strokes of the lung" [18, 19].

2. Pharmacological treatment in stable COPD

The main goals for the management of stable COPD are improvement in quality of life by relieving symptoms and increasing exercise tolerance and reduction of mortality risk by preventing exacerbations and disease progression [1].

Several inhaled, oral, and systemically administered drugs improve lung function, decrease the frequency and severity of COPD exacerbations, and improve patients' quality of life [20].

Non-pharmacological therapies in COPD, including smoking cessation strategies, pulmonary rehabilitation, vaccinations, surgical or bronchoscopic interventions, and noninvasive ventilation have their established role in the management of the disease; however they are not discussed here, as the focus of this chapter is on the pharmacological treatment.

Back in 2001 when the first edition of the GOLD document was released [21], the pharmacological arsenal for the treatment of COPD was rather limited, comprising of short-acting beta2-agonists and anticholinergics, long-acting beta2-agonists, theophyllines, and mucoactive agents. Inhaled corticosteroids, although available as single medication, were never widely recommended for the treatment of COPD in monotherapy and have no current authorization for use outside fixed-dose combinations.

Nowadays, there is a broader range of molecules recommended for the treatment of stable COPD that can be classified in the following classes of pharmacological agents:

- Beta2-agonists: short-acting (SABA) and long-acting (LABA)
- Anticholinergics: short-acting (SAMA) and long-acting (LAMA)
- Fixed-dose combinations: SABA/SAMA, LABA/ICS, LABA/LAMA, LABA/LAMA/ICS
- Methylxanthines
- Phosphodiesterase-4 (PDE4) inhibitors
- Mucolytics
- Antibiotics

Additionally, a new acquisition in the bronchodilator portfolio could be the potential use of dual agents or bifunctional muscarinic antagonists and beta2-agonists (MABAs), which combine both antimuscarinic and adrenergic properties in a single molecule [22]. Some of these molecules are already in clinical trials, but a major caveat is the difficulty to balance the antimuscarinic and adrenergic activities, without expressing a tendency toward one of them [23].

Efforts have been made for the discovery of new pharmacological agents, either belonging to the mentioned classes or addressing new therapeutic targets: new corticosteroids, novel classes of bronchodilators, kinase inhibitors, mediator antagonists (including biological therapies, such as cytokine inhibitors), antioxidants, etc. Unfortunately, many of these molecules never made it to the market or were not granted approval for COPD due to safety, efficacy, or delivery issues; several others are still in the development process [23].

Currently available pharmacological agents and other therapies are mainly used as pathogenic or symptomatic treatment.

2.1 Improvement of lung function and symptoms

Chronic airflow limitation is a central characteristic of COPD and is the result of the combination in varying degrees of several pathological processes such as narrowing of the airways, mucus hypersecretion, and loss of small conducting airways [24]. The consequences of these anatomic changes are expiratory airflow limitation, air trapping, and ventilation-perfusion mismatch [22, 25]. Additionally, the loss of elastic recoil and hyperinflation adversely affect thoracic and diaphragmatic mechanics, increasing the work of breathing and ultimately leading to dynamic hyperinflation [26]. Hyperinflation is an independent predictor of mortality in COPD [27].

The clinical expression of airflow limitation is chronic, progressive dyspnea, which typically worsens with physical exercise. Chronic cough with or without sputum production is usually a reflection of the ongoing inflammatory process in the airways of COPD patients. However, there is no linear correlation between the severity of the airflow limitation and the level of symptoms. Some patients may have little subjective complaints, although the lung function testing reveals various degrees of airflow limitation, while other patients may have significant complaints, with little or no evidence of airflow obstruction [28]. In some cases, the symptoms may precede the development of airflow limitation by many years [1].

Treatment with inhaled bronchodilators can reduce hyperinflation, improve dyspnea, and increase exercise tolerance [29], and therefore, bronchodilators are considered as a cornerstone in the management of stable COPD [30].

While short-acting bronchodilators are an option for patients with occasional dyspnea at low risk of exacerbations, the majority of patients have breathlessness leading to exercise limitation at the time of diagnosis and may require more intensive treatment than short-acting bronchodilators alone [30]. For these patients, whether or not they are also at higher risk of exacerbations, long-acting bronchodilators (as monotherapy or in combination) are recommended as a preferred treatment choice in the GOLD strategy report [1].

Airway tone is controlled by both the sympathetic and parasympathetic nervous systems. These mechanisms interact and may potentiate each other and are employed alone or in combination therapeutically. Relaxation of airway smooth muscle is caused by blockade of acetylcholine activity at the receptor (muscarinic antagonist) or stimulation of the G protein-coupled receptor (beta-agonist) [31].

Anticholinergic drugs in the form of smoked alkaloids were among the first effective treatments for asthma [32]. In the mid-twentieth century, parenteral muscarinic antagonists and beta-agonists were used for acute attacks of asthma [33]. The major disadvantages of the systemic delivery were the side effects and a short duration of benefit. As such, subsequent work has both optimized the receptor specificity and the duration of action [22].

Beta-agonists were in use in Chinese medicine for millennia in the form of ephedra. Developments in the mid-twentieth century yielded compounds that specifically target the beta2-adrenergic receptor, reducing the side effects from beta1-agonists [31].

Since the approval by the US Food and Drug Administration (FDA) in 2004 of the first LAMA, tiotropium, long-acting bronchodilators have begun to play a central role in the management of stable COPD. Currently available molecules for inhalation delivery are summarized in **Table 1**.

The benefits of long-acting bronchodilator monotherapy have been well proven across a range of clinical studies [30] and include improvement of the airflow limitation [34–39], dyspnea [34, 35, 39], physical activity/exercise capacity [29, 40–42], health status [34, 35, 37–39], and prevention of exacerbations [35, 39, 43, 44]; however, many patients remain symptomatic despite treatment [45].

Dual bronchodilation improves lung function compared with a single bronchodilator [30]. Long-acting beta2-agonists and long-acting muscarinic antagonists act via different mechanisms; when used together in patients with COPD, they exert additional bronchodilating effects [46]. Multiple studies have assessed [30] and demonstrated that the use of LABA/LAMA dual bronchodilation results in additional improvements in lung function, exacerbation rates, health status, and other outcome measures when compared with monobronchodilation, while the safety profile of the dual bronchodilators was similar to that observed with placebo and individual monocomponents. Currently available LABA/LAMA combinations are listed in **Table 2**.

According to current guidelines and strategy reports, long-acting bronchodilators in monotherapy are adequate options for the majority of COPD patients, regardless of the disease severity. However, in the GOLD report 2019 [1], the authors provide a clarification of the concept of "escalation" and "de-escalation" of the COPD therapy, which was introduced in a previous version. While "de-escalation" is mainly employed for the withdrawal of ICS due to lack of response or

	Delivery type	Duration of action (h)
Long-acting beta2-agonists (LABA)		
Arformoterol	Nebulized	12
Formoterol	DPI	12
Indacaterol	DPI	24
Olodaterol	SMI	24
Salmeterol	MDI, DPI	12
Long-acting anticholinergics (LAMA)		
Aclidinium bromide	DPI, MDI	12
Glycopyrronium bromide	DPI	12–24
Tiotropium	DPI, SMI	24
Umeclidinium	DPI	24

DPI = dry powder inhaler; MDI = metered dose inhaler; SMI = soft mist inhaler.

Table 1.
Currently available LABAs and LAMAs as monotherapy.

	Delivery type	Duration of action (h)
Fixed-dose combinations of LABA and LAMA (LABA/LAMA)		
Formoterol/Aclidinium	DPI	12
Formoterol/Glycopyrronium	MDI	12
Indacaterol/Glycopyrronium	DPI	12–24
Olodaterol/Tiotropium	SMI	24
Vilanterol/Umeclidinium	DPI	24

DPI = dry powder inhaler; MDI = metered dose inhaler; SMI = soft mist inhaler.

Table 2.
Currently available fixed-dose combinations of LABA/LAMA.

side effects, such as pneumonia, the "escalation" of treatment should be prompted by either inappropriate symptomatic response to the initial therapy or by the presence of exacerbations despite regular treatment and consists of adding a second class of bronchodilator and/or an ICS and/or other pharmacological agents (azithromycin, roflumilast) in order to ensure maximal symptom relief and to curb the risk of exacerbations.

The choice of the bronchodilator treatment should take into account several factors, such as physiological impairment, symptom burden, and exacerbation risk, and should be individualized according to the drug safety profile, cost, and patients' preference for device and medication [1, 20].

One of the current controversies in COPD [20] is the following: what is best, a progressive escalation of bronchodilator therapy or "maximizing" bronchodilator therapy with dual bronchodilator therapy ab initio? The members of the GOLD Scientific Committee suggest that ensuring a maximal bronchodilation from the beginning could be a reasonable approach for both patients with high symptom burden and patients less severely affected. The latter may underreport their symptoms, masking an underlying resting and exercise lung hyperinflation, which is further linked to increased mortality and risk of severe exacerbations [20]. However, if a single agent is preferred, currently available evidence supports the use of a LAMA (tiotropium) since it improves lung function and health status even in patients with milder disease [47].

2.2 Prevention of exacerbations

COPD exacerbations represent acute worsening of symptoms requiring changes in medication and/or hospitalization [1]. Anthonisen and colleagues' criteria [48] have been used for decades now in an attempt to standardize the evaluation of these events; however COPD exacerbations still have no universally established definition [49] and are subject to diagnostic uncertainty [50].

Historically, the level of healthcare resource use (HCRU) required for the management of COPD exacerbations was used both to define and quantify the severity of the exacerbations, with moderate exacerbations requiring administration of oral steroids and/or antibiotics and severe exacerbations requiring hospitalization [49, 51–53]. However, healthcare use in COPD varies widely depending on access, leading to disparities across different healthcare systems [54]. Furthermore, in order to be treated, an acute event should be reported to healthcare professionals; hence unreported events may not be captured by HCRU definitions. In some reports, such events comprise up to two-thirds of exacerbations and can impair health-related quality of life [55, 56] and increase the risk of hospitalization [57].

Another approach to define exacerbations is based on the systematic and standardized assessment of daily symptoms recorded using specific questionnaires (diaries) administered to the patients on paper or electronically. These questionnaires were developed with the ability to detect worsening of symptoms beyond a pre-specified threshold, based on patients' reporting of their daily symptoms [58, 59]. Advantages of a standardized, validated assessment of COPD symptoms in exacerbation studies include uniform metrics, reduced recall bias, and the ability to fully characterize exacerbations of COPD, including the estimated 50–70% of events that are unreported [55, 56, 59]. Although attractive, this kind of approach is more difficult to implement outside the clinical trial setting, and the concordance with the HCRU-defined events is modest [54, 60].

COPD exacerbations have a marked negative effect on both the patient and underlying disease processes [61] and can result in hospitalization and readmission, an increased risk of death [62], and a significant reduction in health status [55]. Exacerbations are also associated with long-term decline in lung function and a high socioeconomic cost [63, 64]. A history of frequent exacerbations is a good predictor for future exacerbation risk and defines the "frequent exacerbator" phenotype [65]. Thus, optimizing the prevention and management of COPD exacerbations are important clinical issues [61].

The GOLD strategy report stratifies COPD patients based on the severity of their airflow limitation, symptom burden, and the risk of exacerbations; however the recommendations for the pharmacological treatment rely exclusively on the level of symptoms and exacerbation risk [1].

While the initial assessment of exacerbation risk may be biased by the patients' ability to recall historical episodes of symptom worsening prior to being diagnosed with COPD, the reassessment of risk after initial pharmacological treatment should be able to identify patients requiring an escalation of treatment for a better prevention of future exacerbation episodes.

The preferred treatment options for patients at high risk of exacerbation are a LAMA in monotherapy, a LABA/LAMA, or a LABA/ICS combination [1].

There is evidence that both LABAs and LAMAs significantly improve the exacerbation rate versus placebo [66–68]; however, clinical trials have shown a greater effect on exacerbation rates for LAMA treatment (tiotropium) versus LABA treatment [69, 70].

There is a strong evidence that treatment with fixed-dose combinations of LABA/LAMA improves lung function, symptoms, and health-related quality of life compared to placebo or its individual bronchodilator components [71–73]. The superiority of dual bronchodilation in the prevention of exacerbations compared to monocomponents was demonstrated for a LABA/LAMA combination [74], while another large study found that combining a LABA with a LAMA did not reduce exacerbation rate as much as expected compared to LAMA alone [75].

Similarly, an ICS combined with a LABA is more effective than the individual components in improving lung function and health status and reducing exacerbations in patients with a history of exacerbations and moderate to very severe COPD [76, 77]. Currently available ICS/LABA combinations are listed in **Table 3**.

Furthermore, another study demonstrated the superiority of a LABA/LAMA combination versus an ICS/LABA combination in the prevention of exacerbations in patients with moderate to very severe COPD and a history of exacerbations, regardless of baseline blood eosinophils [78].

In a recently published review, a group of experts critically evaluated mechanisms potentially responsible for the increased benefit of LABA/LAMA combinations over single long-acting bronchodilators or LABA/inhaled corticosteroids in decreasing exacerbation. These included effects on lung hyperinflation and

	Delivery type	Duration of action (h)
Fixed-dose combinations of LABA and ICS (LABA/ICS)		
Formoterol/Beclometasone	MDI	12
Formoterol/Budesonide	MDI, DPI	12
Formoterol/Mometasone	MDI	12
Salmeterol/Fluticasone	MDI, DPI	12
Vilanterol/Fluticasone furoate	DPI	24

DPI = dry powder inhaler; MDI = metered dose inhaler.

Table 3.
Currently available fixed-dose combinations of LABA/ICS.

	Delivery type	Duration of action (h)
Fixed-dose combinations of LABA, LAMA and ICS (LABA/LAMA/ICS)		
Formoterol/Glycopyrronium/Beclometasone	MDI	12
Vilanterol/Umeclidinium/Fluticasone furoate	DPI	24
Formoterol/Glycopyrronium/Budesonide	MDI	12

DPI = dry powder inhaler; MDI = metered dose inhaler.

Table 4.
Currently available fixed-dose combinations of LABA/LAMA/ICS.

mechanical stress, inflammation, excessive mucus production with impaired mucociliary clearance, and symptom severity [79].

Although triple therapy in separate inhalers is already in use for COPD patients for a couple of years now, fixed triple therapy combining an ICS, a LABA, and a LAMA in a single inhaler recently emerged on the market. Currently, there are only two products approved by the European Medicines Agency (EMA) for use in COPD, and a third one was recently approved in Japan (see **Table 4**) [80].

Several recent studies have demonstrated that single-inhaler triple therapy is more effective in reducing the exacerbation than LAMA alone, a LABA/ICS, or a LABA/LAMA combination [81–84].

The GOLD algorithm for the escalation of treatment in patients with persistent risk of exacerbations despite regular treatment provides that patients taking a single bronchodilator should be switched to dual bronchodilation and then to triple therapy and/or additional therapies. Alternatively, some patients with high blood eosinophils may benefit from a LABA/ICS combination prior to receiving triple therapy [1].

The use of ICS in COPD has become very controversial in the last years, owing on the one hand to the limited effect on lung function and on the other hand to potential side effects associated with long-term use at the higher doses recommended for the treatment of COPD. These include:

- Risk of infections such as pneumonia [85], tuberculosis and non-tuberculous mycobacterial disease [86], and oropharyngeal candidiasis [87]

- Skin lesions [88]

- Diabetes onset and progression [89]

- Increased risk of bone fractures [90]
- Cataracts [91]

The use of ICS alone is discouraged in COPD [20]; however several studies have demonstrated a consistent effect on exacerbation reduction of LABA/ICS fixed-dose combinations versus individual monocomponents [76, 77, 87, 92, 93].

The need for biomarkers accurately assessing disease activity and response to therapy in order to develop better COPD treatment is well acknowledged [94]. Peripheral blood eosinophil level has emerged in the recent years as a promising biomarker, showing capabilities to predict both the risk of exacerbation and the magnitude of response to ICS therapy [95–97]. Thus, several post hoc or pre-specified analyses of clinical trials have shown that blood eosinophil levels may indicate which patients can benefit from a reduction of exacerbations by the treatment with ICS-containing regimens [84, 96, 98]. Various cutoff points were proposed for the level of blood eosinophils in order to identify the patients who would benefit most from the ICS therapy. A recent pooled analysis (n = 4528) evidenced that a level of blood eosinophils >300/mmc^3 suggests a beneficial role of ICS, while a low level of blood eosinophils (<100/mmc^3) may be a negative predictor of the ICS effects. This was previously observed in other two post hoc analyses [99, 100] and was confirmed in a pre-specified analysis of another randomized clinical trial [101].

Other classes of pharmacological agents, such as PDE4-inhibitors (roflumilast) or antibiotics (azithromycin) administered orally on top of inhaled therapy, may bring an additional benefit in reducing exacerbations [102, 103]. The side effects, however, limit their use to selected patients only.

2.3 Mortality risk

Two large clinical trials have failed to demonstrate a positive effect of the active treatments (LABA/ICS, ICS alone, and LABA alone) versus placebo on the mortality risk [36, 104].

Smoking cessation, vaccinations, supplemental oxygen for hypoxemic patients, and lung volume reduction surgery in selected patients are the only therapies that have been proven to improve survival; smoking cessation also attenuates disease progression [20].

3. Conclusions

Inhaled long-acting bronchodilator treatment plays a central role in the management of stable COPD. Anti-inflammatory treatment with inhaled corticosteroids in combination with a long-acting beta2 agonist or with dual bronchodilation (LABA and LAMA) as part of the triple therapy improves outcomes especially in patients with high blood eosinophil level.

Despite all the progress made in the recent years in the field of COPD, we are still lacking drugs that can effectively modify the course of the disease [23].

The unmet needs in COPD warrant further research for the discovery of new biomarkers and effective therapeutic agents able to radically improve short-term and long-term outcomes in patients suffering of this disease.

Author details

Stefan-Marian Frent
Department of Pulmonology, University of Medicine and Pharmacy Timisoara, Timisoara, Romania

*Address all correspondence to: frentz.stefan@umft.ro

References

[1] Singh D, Agusti A, Anzueto A, Barnes PJ, et al. Global strategy for the diagnosis, management, and prevention of chronic obstructive lung disease: The GOLD science committee report 2019. The European Respiratory Journal. 2019;**53**(5):pii: 1900164. DOI: 10.1183/13993003.00164-2019

[2] Lozano R, Naghavi M, Foreman K, et al. Global and regional mortality from 235 causes of death for 20 age groups in 1990 and 2010: A systematic analysis for the global burden of disease study 2010. Lancet. 2012;**380**(9859):2095-2128

[3] Vos T, Flaxman AD, Naghavi M, et al. Years lived with disability (YLDs) for 1160 sequelae of 289 diseases and injuries 1990–2010: A systematic analysis for the Global Burden of Disease Study 2010. Lancet. 2012; **380**(9859):2163-2196

[4] Adeloye D, Chua S, Lee C, et al. Global and regional estimates of COPD prevalence: Systematic review and meta-analysis. Journal of Global Health. 2015;**5**:020415

[5] Mathers CD, Loncar D. Projections of global mortality and burden of disease from 2002 to 2030. PLoS Medicine. 2006;**3**(11):e442

[6] Stoller JK, Aboussouan LS. Alpha1-antitrypsin deficiency. Lancet. 2005; **365**(9478):2225-2236

[7] McCloskey SC, Patel BD, Hinchliffe SJ, Reid ED, Wareham NJ, Lomas DA. Siblings of patients with severe chronic obstructive pulmonary disease have a significant risk of airflow obstruction. American Journal of Respiratory and Critical Care Medicine. 2001;**164**(8 Pt 1):1419-1424

[8] Eisner MD, Anthonisen M, Coultas D, et al. An official American Thoracic Society public policy statement: Novel risk factors and the global burden of chronic obstructive pulmonary disease. American Journal of Respiratory and Critical Care Medicine. 2010;**182**(5):693-718

[9] Ezzati M. Indoor air pollution and health in developing countries. Lancet. 2005;**366**(9480):104-106

[10] Assad NA, Balmes J, Mehta S, Cheema U, Sood A. Chronic obstructive pulmonary disease secondary to household air pollution. Seminars in Respiratory and Critical Care Medicine. 2015;**36**(3):408-421

[11] Liu S, Zhou Y, Liu S, et al. Association between exposure to ambient particulate matter and chronic obstructive pulmonary disease: Results from a cross-sectional study in China. Thorax. 2017;**72**(9):788-795

[12] Balmes J, Becklake M, Blanc P, et al. American Thoracic Society statement: Occupational contribution to the burden of airway disease. American Journal of Respiratory and Critical Care Medicine. 2003;**167**(5):787-797

[13] Bigna JJ, Kenne AM, Asangbeh SL, Sibetcheu AT. Prevalence of chronic obstructive pulmonary disease in the global population with HIV: A systematic review and meta-analysis. The Lancet Global Health. 2018;**6**(2): e193-e202

[14] Byrne AL, Marais BJ, Mitnick CD, Lecca L, Marks GB. Tuberculosis and chronic respiratory disease: A systematic review. International Journal of Infectious Diseases. 2015;**32**:138-146

[15] Townend J, Minelli C, Mortimer K, et al. The association between chronic airflow obstruction and poverty in 12 sites of the multinational BOLD study.

The European Respiratory Journal. 2017; **49**(6):pii: 1601880

[16] GBD 2013 DALYs and HALE Collaborators, Murray CJ, Barber RM, et al. Global, regional, and national disability-adjusted life years (DALYs) for 306 diseases and injuries and healthy life expectancy (HALE) for 188 countries, 1990–2013: Quantifying the epidemiological transition. Lancet. 2015; **386**(10009):2145-2191

[17] Halpin DM, Decramer M, Celli B, Kesten S, Liu D, Tashkin DP. Exacerbation frequency and course of COPD. International Journal of Chronic Obstructive Pulmonary Disease. 2012;**7**: 653-661

[18] Celli BR. Dissecting COPD exacerbations: Time to rethink our definition. The European Respiratory Journal. 2017;**50**:1701432

[19] Hillas G, Perlikos F, Tzanakis N. Acute exacerbation of COPD: Is it the "stroke of the lungs"? International Journal of Chronic Obstructive Pulmonary Disease. 2016;**11**:1579-1586

[20] Criner GJ, Martinez FJ, et al. Current controversies in chronic obstructive pulmonary disease. A report from the Global Initiative for Chronic Obstructive Lung Disease Scientific Committee. Annals of the American Thoracic Society. 2019;**16**(1):29-39

[21] Pauwels RA, Buist AS, Calverley PM, Jenkins CR, Hurd SS, GOLD Scientific Committee. Global strategy for the diagnosis, management, and prevention of chronic obstructive pulmonary disease. NHLBI/WHO Global Initiative For Chronic Obstructive Lung Disease (GOLD) Workshop summary. American Journal of Respiratory and Critical Care Medicine. 2001;**163**(5):1256-1276

[22] Cohen JS, Miles MC, Donohue JF, Ohar JA. Dual therapy strategies for COPD: The scientific rationale for LAMA + LABA. International Journal of Chronic Obstructive Pulmonary Disease. 2016;**11**:785-797

[23] Gross NJ, Barnes PJ. New therapies for asthma and chronic obstructive pulmonary disease. American Journal of Respiratory and Critical Care Medicine. 2017;**195**(2):159-166

[24] McDonough JE, Yuan R, Suzuki M, et al. Small-airway obstruction and emphysema in chronic obstructive pulmonary disease. The New England Journal of Medicine. 2011;**365**(17): 1567-1575

[25] Senior R, Atkinson J. Chronic obstructive pulmonary disease: Epidemiology, pathophysiology, and pathogenesis. In: Alfred Fishman M, editor. Fishman's Pulmonary Diseases and Disorders. 4th ed. Vol. 1. New York, NY: McGraw Hill Medical; 2008. pp. 707-728

[26] O'Donnell DE, Laveneziana P. Physiology and consequences of lung hyperinflation in COPD. European Respiratory Review. 2006;**15**(100): 61-67

[27] Casanova C, Cote C, de Torres JP, et al. Inspiratory-to-total lung capacity ratio predicts mortality in patients with chronic obstructive pulmonary disease. American Journal of Respiratory and Critical Care Medicine. 2005;**171**(6): 591-597

[28] Montes de Oca M, Perez-Padilla R, Talamo C, et al. Acute bronchodilator responsiveness in subjects with and without airflow obstruction in five Latin American cities: The PLATINO study. Pulmonary Pharmacology & Therapeutics. 2010;**23**(1):29-35

[29] O'Donnell DE, Fluge T, Gerken F, et al. Effects of tiotropium on lung hyperinflation, dyspnoea and exercise

tolerance in COPD. The European Respiratory Journal. 2004;**23**(6):832-840

[30] Thomas M, Halpin D, Miravitlles M. When is dual bronchodilation indicated in COPD? International Journal of Chronic Obstructive Pulmonary Disease. 2017;**12**:2291-2305

[31] Cazzola M, Page CP, Calzetta L, Matera MG. Pharmacology and therapeutics of bronchodilators. Pharmacological Reviews. 2012;**64**(3): 450-504

[32] Jackson M. "Divine stramonium": The rise and fall of smoking for asthma. Medical History. 2010;**54**(2):171-194

[33] Bray GW. The treatment of asthma. British Medical Journal. 1935;**1**(3863): 119-121

[34] Donohue JF, van Noord JA, Bateman ED, et al. A 6-month, placebo-controlled study comparing lung function and health status changes in COPD patients treated with tiotropium or salmeterol. Chest. 2002;**122**(1):47-55

[35] D'Urzo A, Ferguson GT, van Noord JA, et al. Efficacy and safety of once-daily NVA237 in patients with moderate-to-severe COPD: The GLOW1 trial. Respiratory Research. 2011;**12**:156

[36] Calverley PM, Anderson JA, Celli B, et al. Salmeterol and fluticasone propionate and survival in chronic obstructive pulmonary disease. The New England Journal of Medicine. 2007; **356**(8):775-789

[37] Rossi A, Kristufek P, Levine BE, et al. Comparison of the efficacy, tolerability, and safety of formoterol dry powder and oral, slow-release theophylline in the treatment of COPD. Chest. 2002;**121**(4):1058-1069

[38] Chapman KR, Rennard SI, Dogra A, et al. Long-term safety and efficacy of indacaterol, a long-acting β2-agonist, in subjects with COPD: A randomized, placebo-controlled study. Chest. 2011; **140**(1):68-75

[39] Kerwin EM, D'Urzo AD, Gelb AF, Lakkis H, Garcia GE, Caracta CF. Efficacy and safety of a 12-week treatment with twice-daily aclidinium bromide in COPD patients (ACCORD COPD I). COPD. 2012;**9**(2):90-101

[40] Beeh KM, Singh D, Di Scala L, Drollmann A. Once-daily NVA237 improves exercise tolerance from the first dose in patients with COPD: The GLOW3 trial. International Journal of Chronic Obstructive Pulmonary Disease. 2012;7:503-513

[41] Maltais F, Celli B, Casaburi R, et al. Aclidinium bromide improves exercise endurance and lung hyperinflation in patients with moderate to severe COPD. Respiratory Medicine. 2011;**105**(4): 580-587

[42] O'Donnell DE, Casaburi R, Vincken W, et al. Effect of indacaterol on exercise endurance and lung hyperinflation in COPD. Respiratory Medicine. 2011;**105**(7):1030-1036

[43] Halpin DM, Vogelmeier C, Pieper MP, Metzdorf N, Richard F, Anzueto A. Effect of tiotropium on COPD exacerbations: A systematic review. Respiratory Medicine. 2016; **114**:1-8

[44] Jones PW, Singh D, Bateman ED, et al. Efficacy and safety of twice-daily aclidinium bromide in COPD patients: The ATTAIN study. The European Respiratory Journal. 2012;**40**(4): 830-836

[45] Price D, West D, Brusselle G, et al. Management of COPD in the UK primary-care setting: An analysis of real-life prescribing patterns. International Journal of Chronic

Obstructive Pulmonary Disease. 2014;**9**: 889-905

[46] Tashkin DP, Ferguson GT. Combination bronchodilator therapy in the management of chronic obstructive pulmonary disease. Respiratory Research. 2013;**14**:49

[47] Zhou Y, Zhong NS, Li X, et al. Tiotropium in early-stage chronic obstructive pulmonary disease. The New England Journal of Medicine. 2017; **377**:923-935

[48] Anthonisen NR, Manfreda J, Warren CP, Hershfield ES, Harding GK, Nelson NA. Antibiotic therapy in exacerbations of chronic obstructive pulmonary disease. Annals of Internal Medicine. 1987;**106**: 196-204

[49] Rodriguez-Roisin R. Toward a consensus definition for COPD exacerbations. Chest. 2000;**117**:398s-401s

[50] Sapey E, Stockley RA. COPD exacerbations. 2: Aetiology. Thorax. 2006;**61**:250-258

[51] Burge S, Wedzicha JA. COPD exacerbations: Definitions and classifications. The European Respiratory Journal. Supplement. 2003; **41**:46s-53s

[52] Calverley P, Pauwels Dagger R, Lofdahl CG, Svensson K, Higenbottam T, Carlsson LG, et al. Relationship between respiratory symptoms and medical treatment in exacerbations of COPD. The European Respiratory Journal. 2005;**26**:406-413

[53] Wedzicha JA, Seemungal TA. COPD exacerbations: Defining their cause and prevention. Lancet. 2007;**370**(9589): 786-796

[54] Frent SM, Chapman KR, et al. Capturing exacerbations of chronic obstructive pulmonary disease with EXACT. A subanalysis of FLAME. American Journal of Respiratory and Critical Care Medicine. 2019;**199**(1): 43-51

[55] Seemungal TA, Donaldson GC, Paul EA, Bestall JC, Jeffries DJ, Wedzicha JA. Effect of exacerbation on quality of life in patients with chronic obstructive pulmonary disease. American Journal of Respiratory and Critical Care Medicine. 1998;**157**: 1418-1422

[56] Langsetmo L, Platt RW, Ernst P, Bourbeau J. Underreporting exacerbation of chronic obstructive pulmonary disease in a longitudinal cohort. American Journal of Respiratory and Critical Care Medicine. 2008;**177**: 396-401

[57] Wilkinson TM, Donaldson GC, Hurst JR, Seemungal TA, Wedzicha JA. Early therapy improves outcomes of exacerbations of chronic obstructive pulmonary disease. American Journal of Respiratory and Critical Care Medicine. 2004;**169**:1298-1303

[58] Kulich K, Keininger DL, Tiplady B, Banerji D. Symptoms and impact of COPD assessed by an electronic diary in patients with moderate-to-severe COPD: Psychometric results from the SHINE study. International Journal of Chronic Obstructive Pulmonary Disease. 2015;**10**:79-94

[59] Leidy NK, Wilcox TK, Jones PW, Murray L, Winnette R, Howard K, et al. Development of the EXAcerbations of chronic obstructive pulmonary disease tool (EXACT): A patient-reported outcome (PRO) measure. Value in Health. 2010;**13**: 965-975

[60] Jones PW, Lamarca R, Chuecos F, Singh D, Agusti A, Bateman ED, et al.

Characterisation and impact of reported and unreported exacerbations: Results from ATTAIN. The European Respiratory Journal. 2014;**44**:1156-1165

[61] Marc Miravitlles M, Anzueto A, Jardim JR. Optimizing bronchodilation in the prevention of COPD exacerbations. Respiratory Research. 2017;**18**(1):125

[62] Soler-Cataluña JJ, Martínez-García MA, Román Sánchez P, Salcedo E, Navarro M, Ochando R. Severe acute exacerbations and mortality in patients with chronic obstructive pulmonary disease. Thorax. 2005;**60**:925-931

[63] Donaldson GC, Seemungal TA, Bhowmik A, Wedzicha JA. Relationship between exacerbation frequency and lung function decline in chronicobstructive pulmonary disease. Thorax. 2002;**57**:847-852

[64] Dhamane AD, Moretz C, Zhou Y, Burslem K, Saverno K, Jain G, et al. COPD exacerbation frequency and its association with health care resource utilization and costs. International Journal of Chronic Obstructive Pulmonary Disease. 2015;**10**: 2609-2618

[65] Hurst JR, Vestbo J, Anzueto A, Locantore N, Müllerova H, Tal-Singer R, et al. Susceptibility to exacerbation in chronic obstructive pulmonary disease. The New England Journal of Medicine. 2010;**363**:1128-1138

[66] Kew KM, Mavergames C, Walters JA. Long-acting beta2-agonists for chronic obstructive pulmonary disease. Cochrane Database of Systematic Reviews. 2013;**10**:CD010177

[67] Geake JB, Dabscheck EJ, Wood-Baker R, Cates CJ. Indacaterol, a once-daily beta2-agonist, versus twice-daily $beta_2$-agonists or placebo for chronic obstructive pulmonary disease. Cochrane Database of Systematic Reviews. 2015;**1**:CD010139

[68] Karner C, Chong J, Poole P. Tiotropium versus placebo for chronic obstructive pulmonary disease. Cochrane Database of Systematic Reviews. 2014;**7**(7):CD009285

[69] Vogelmeier C, Hederer B, Glaab T, et al. Tiotropium versus salmeterol for the prevention of exacerbations of COPD. The New England Journal of Medicine. 2011;**364**(12):1093-1103

[70] Decramer ML, Chapman KR, Dahl R, et al. Once-daily indacaterol versus tiotropium for patients with severe chronic obstructive pulmonary disease (INVIGORATE): A randomised, blinded, parallel-group study. The Lancet Respiratory Medicine. 2013;**1**(7): 524-533

[71] Mahler DA, Decramer M, D'Urzo A, et al. Dual bronchodilation with QVA149 reduces patient-reported dyspnoea in COPD: The BLAZE study. The European Respiratory Journal. 2014;**43**(6):1599-1609

[72] Singh D, Ferguson GT, Bolitschek J, et al. Tiotropium + olodaterol shows clinically meaningful improvements in quality of life. Respiratory Medicine. 2015;**109**(10):1312-1319

[73] Bateman ED, Chapman KR, Singh D, et al. Aclidinium bromide and formoterol fumarate as a fixed-dose combination in COPD: Pooled analysis of symptoms and exacerbations from two six-month, multicentre, randomised studies (ACLIFORM and AUGMENT). Respiratory Research. 2015;**16**:92

[74] Wedzicha JA, Decramer M, Ficker JH, et al. Analysis of chronic obstructive pulmonary disease exacerbations with the dual bronchodilator QVA149 compared with glycopyrronium and tiotropium

(SPARK): A randomised, double-blind, parallel-group study. The Lancet Respiratory Medicine. 2013;**1**(3): 199-209

[75] Calverley PMA, Anzueto AR, Carter K, et al. Tiotropium and olodaterol in the prevention of chronic obstructive pulmonary disease exacerbations (DYNAGITO): A double-blind, randomised, parallel-group, active-controlled trial. The Lancet Respiratory Medicine. 2018;**6**(5): 337-344

[76] Nannini LJ, Lasserson TJ, Poole P. Combined corticosteroid and long-acting beta(2)-agonist in one inhaler versus long-acting beta(2)-agonists for chronic obstructive pulmonary disease. Cochrane Database of Systematic Reviews. 2012;**9**(9):CD006829

[77] Nannini LJ, Poole P, Milan SJ, Kesterton A. Combined corticosteroid and long-acting beta(2)-agonist in one inhaler versus inhaled corticosteroids alone for chronic obstructive pulmonary disease. Cochrane Database of Systematic Reviews. 2013;**8**(8): CD006826

[78] Wedzicha JA, Banerji D, Chapman KR, et al. Indacaterol-glycopyrronium versus salmeterol-fluticasone for COPD. The New England Journal of Medicine. 2016;**374**(23): 2222-2234

[79] Beeh KM, Burgel PR, Franssen FME, et al. How do dual long-acting bronchodilators prevent exacerbations of chronic obstructive pulmonary disease? American Journal of Respiratory and Critical Care Medicine. 2017;**196**(2):139-149

[80] AstraZeneca. Breztri Aerosphere (PT010) Approved in Japan for Patients with Chronic Obstructive Pulmonary Disease [Internet]. 2019. Available from: https://www.astrazeneca.com/media-centre/press-releases/2019/breztri-aerosphere-pt010-approved-in-japan-for-patients-with-chronic-obstructive-pulmonary-disease-19062019.html [Accessed: September 18, 2019]

[81] Vestbo J, Papi A, Corradi M, et al. Single inhaler extrafine triple therapy versus long-acting muscarinic antagonist therapy for chronic obstructive pulmonary disease (TRINITY): A double-blind, parallel group, randomised controlled trial. Lancet. 2017;**389**(10082):1919-1929

[82] Singh D, Papi A, Corradi M, et al. Single inhaler triple therapy versus inhaled corticosteroid plus long-acting β2-agonist therapy for chronic obstructive pulmonary disease (TRILOGY): A double-blind, parallel group, randomised controlled trial. Lancet. 2016;**388**:963-973

[83] Papi A, Vestbo J, Fabbri L, et al. Extrafine inhaled triple therapy versus dual bronchodilator therapy in chronic obstructive pulmonary disease (TRIBUTE): A double-blind, parallel group, randomised controlled trial. Lancet. 2018;**391**(10125):1076-1084

[84] Lipson DA, Barnhart F, Brealey N, et al. Once-daily single-inhaler triple versus dual therapy in patients with COPD. The New England Journal of Medicine. 2018;**378**(18):1671-1680

[85] Kew KM, Seniukovich A. Inhaled steroids and risk of pneumonia for chronic obstructive pulmonary disease. Cochrane Database of Systematic Reviews. 2014;**10**:CD010115

[86] Brode SK, Campitelli MA, Kwong JC, et al. The risk of mycobacterial infections associated with inhaled corticosteroid use. The European Respiratory Journal. 2017;**50**: pii: 1700037

[87] Dransfield MT, Bourbeau J, Jones PW, et al. Once-daily inhaled fluticasone furoate and vilanterol versus

vilanterol only for prevention of exacerbations of COPD: Two replicate double-blind, parallel-group, randomised controlled trials. The Lancet Respiratory Medicine. 2013;**1**:210-223

[88] Price D, Yawn B, Brusselle G, Rossi A. Risk-to-benefit ratio of inhaled corticosteroids in patients with COPD. Primary Care Respiratory Journal. 2013; **22**:92-100

[89] Suissa S, Kezouh A, Ernst P. Inhaled corticosteroids and the risks of diabetes onset and progression. The American Journal of Medicine. 2010;**123**: 1001-1006

[90] Gonzalez AV, Coulombe J, Ernst P, Suissa S. Long-term use of inhaled corticosteroids in COPD and the risk of fracture. Chest. 2017;**153**(2):321-328

[91] Cumming RG, Mitchell P, Leeder SR. Use of inhaled corticosteroids and the risk of cataracts. The New England Journal of Medicine. 1997;**337**(1):8-14

[92] Calverley P, Pauwels R, Vestbo J, et al. Combined salmeterol and fluticasone in the treatment of chronic obstructive pulmonary disease: A randomised controlled trial. Lancet. 2003;**361**:449-456

[93] Sharafkhaneh A, Southard JG, Goldman M, Uryniak T, Martin UJ. Effect of budesonide/formoterol pMDI on COPD exacerbations: A double-blind, randomized study. Respiratory Medicine. 2012;**106**(2):257-268

[94] Mannino DM. Biomarkers in COPD: The search continues! The European Respiratory Journal. 2015;**45**:872-874

[95] Vedel-Krogh S, Nielsen SF, Lange P, Vestbo J, Nordestgaard BG. Blood eosinophils and exacerbations in chronic obstructive pulmonary disease. The Copenhagen general population study. American Journal of Respiratory and Critical Care Medicine. 2016;**193**: 965-974

[96] Pascoe S, Locantore N, Dransfield MT, Barnes NC, Pavord ID. Blood eosinophil counts, exacerbations, and response to the addition of inhaled fluticasone furoate to vilanterol in patients with chronic obstructive pulmonary disease: A secondary analysis of data from two parallel randomised controlled trials. The Lancet Respiratory Medicine. 2015;**3**(6):435-442

[97] Bafadhel M, Peterson S, De Blas MA, et al. Predictors of exacerbation risk and response to budesonide in patients with chronic obstructive pulmonary disease: A post-hoc analysis of three randomised trials. The Lancet Respiratory Medicine. 2018; **6**(2):117-126

[98] Siddiqui SH, Guasconi A, Vestbo J, Jones P, Agusti A, Paggiaro P, et al. Blood eosinophils: A biomarker of response to extrafine beclomethasone/formoterol in chronic obstructive pulmonary disease. American Journal of Respiratory and Critical Care Medicine. 2015;**192**:523-525

[99] Watz H, Tetzlaff K, Wouters EF, et al. Blood eosinophil count and exacerbations in severe chronic obstructive pulmonary disease after withdrawal of inhaled corticosteroids: A post-hoc analysis of the WISDOM trial. The Lancet Respiratory Medicine. 2016; **4**:390-398

[100] Roche N, Chapman KR, Vogelmeier CF, et al. Blood eosinophils and response to maintenance chronic obstructive pulmonary disease treatment. Data from the FLAME Trial. American Journal of Respiratory and Critical Care Medicine. 2017;**195**:1189-1197

[101] Chapman KR, Hurst JR, Frent SM, et al. Long-term triple therapy de-escalation to indacaterol/ glycopyrronium in patients with chronic

obstructive pulmonary disease (SUNSET): A randomized, double-blind, triple-dummy clinical trial. American Journal of Respiratory and Critical Care Medicine. 2018;**198**(3):329-339

[102] Calverley PM, Rabe KF, Goehring UM, et al. Roflumilast in symptomatic chronic obstructive pulmonary disease: Two randomised clinical trials. Lancet. 2009;**374**(9691):685-694

[103] Uzun S, Djamin RS, Kluytmans JA, et al. Azithromycin maintenance treatment in patients with frequent exacerbations of chronic obstructive pulmonary disease (COLUMBUS): A randomised, double-blind, placebo-controlled trial. The Lancet Respiratory Medicine. 2014;**2**(5):361-368

[104] Vestbo J, Anderson JA, Brook RD, et al. Fluticasone furoate and vilanterol and survival in chronic obstructive pulmonary disease with heightened cardiovascular risk (SUMMIT): A double-blind randomised controlled trial. Lancet. 2016;**387**(10030):1817-1826

Section 2

Tuberculosis

Chapter 5

Thoracic Extrapulmonary Tuberculosis in the Millennial Era

Onix J. Cantres-Fonseca

Abstract

Mycobacterium tuberculosis is one of the most pathogenic infectious organisms, usually known for causing cavitary lung infection. But this mycobacterium is also capable of causing masked involvement in any organ of the body. Its clinical manifestation can mimic other conditions according to the organ affected. Extrapulmonary infection is defined as any manifestation caused by tuberculosis in tissues outside the airway or the pulmonary parenchyma. Despite it being a well-known infectious organism throughout decades, tuberculosis continues to be causing great morbidity and mortality in this millennium. This chapter will discuss the clinical manifestations of extrapulmonary tuberculosis (EPTB), when the mycobacteria invade extrapulmonary tissues inside the thorax. We discuss and review the literature about the clinical manifestations, diagnosis and evaluation, and general treatment.

Keywords: tuberculosis, extrapulmonary, thoracic

1. Introduction

Mycobacterium tuberculosis is one of the most pathogenic infectious organisms. As a single agent, it has caused more morbidity and mortality around the world than any other organism, despite being known for years and the emergence of effective antibiotic therapy. The most common form of active disease is pulmonary parenchymal involvement. However, with the emergence of longer life expectancy of immunosuppressed patients with human immunodeficiency virus and cancer, these mycobacteria have shown its pathogenicity causing infection outside the lungs, involving a great variability of extrapulmonary tissue and other organ systems.

Extrapulmonary tuberculosis (EPTB) occurs when the tuberculous mycobacterium invades areas outside the pulmonary parenchyma, including other thoracic structures, and any other organ outside the lungs. Cases of extrapulmonary tuberculosis have been reported involving organs from the central nervous system throughout the abdominal organs and even the bone and skin. Clinical presentation will vary according to the organ involved, and its pathogenicity can mimic other infectious and noninfectious diseases. Extrapulmonary infection can be fatal and often requires extensive work-up for proper diagnosis. It often requires invasive interventions as culture of sterile body fluids and biopsies, for evaluation of pathognomonic changes and identification of the mycobacteria. Also, the diagnosis is time-consuming, and delay in identification can occur due to its variable clinical presentation.

Outside the pulmonary parenchyma, tuberculosis can invade any structure of the thorax, causing significant clinical disease. Involvement of any thoracic tissue, outside the airways and alveoli, is considered an extrapulmonary disease. Thoracic extrapulmonary tuberculosis includes involvement of the pleural tissue, the lymph nodes, the heart and blood vessels, the bone and skin, and even the complete chest wall. Also, tuberculosis can cause significant disease if it reaches the thoracic spine. This illustrates the ample spectrum of the pathology of this mycobacterium when it invades tissue outside the lung. Many times, therapy for thoracic extrapulmonary tuberculosis is similar to exclusive pulmonary involvement. However, the fact that extrapulmonary tuberculosis can mimic other diseases, identification of this mycobacteria as the culprit of a thoracic pathology, requires a vast knowledge to include it in the differential diagnosis. Also, thoracic extrapulmonary tuberculosis would require additional diagnostic and therapeutic interventions during patient's management.

In this chapter, we will discuss the most important clinical manifestations of thoracic extrapulmonary tuberculosis. It will include the most common clinical presentations, and a review of the literature is its diagnostic and therapeutic approach.

2. Pathophysiology of thoracic extrapulmonary tuberculosis

The most common presentation thoracic extrapulmonary tuberculosis is lymphadenitis [1]. When the mycobacterium is inhaled into the lungs, it is engulfed by macrophages that activate specific T cells that protect the organism causing mostly latent infection. The lung natural immunity creates a granuloma around infected alveolar macrophages where the mycobacteria can be dormant or can proliferate. Depending of the bacterial load and inflammatory host response, some patients cannot contain the infection in the granulomas, leading to mycobacterial proliferation outside the granulomas, causing active disease [2]. The mycobacteria can also escape the lung throughout blood vessels and the lymphatic system invading other organs. In the same way, mycobacteria can invade extensively the alveolar spaces and reach extrapulmonary tissues after rupture of caseous foci in the proximity [3].

It is thought that most of the extrapulmonary tuberculosis occurs during primary infection rather than reactivation [4–6], especially tuberculous pleurisy [1]. However, in the immunosuppressed population, other extrapulmonary findings are more common after activation of latent disease [2].

3. Epidemiology of thoracic extrapulmonary tuberculosis

When we talk about extrapulmonary tuberculosis, we refer to any invasion of the mycobacteria outside the pulmonary tissue. Invasion of the pleura, thoracic lymph nodes, and structures of the chest wall is part of the spectrum of extrapulmonary disease.

The most common extraparenchymal invasion of the mycobacteria in the thorax is invasion of the supraclavicular, mediastinal, and hilar lymph nodes [1]. Depending of the world location and endemicity of the infection, lymph node infection has been identified between 8 and 30% of the patients [1]. Almost 30% of those patients present with concomitant extra nodal disease [1]. Variability in diagnosis techniques and available resources must probably influence in the lymph node infection being underdiagnosed.

Tuberculous pleural involvement is the second most frequent thoracic extrapulmonary manifestation. Almost 25% of patients with tuberculosis present with pleuritis. The incidence is higher in immunosuppressed patients secondary to human immunodeficiency virus [7]. The incidence of tuberculous pleural involvement can be higher, but its epidemiological data is limited based on world location, patient population, and diagnostic resources. Pleural fluid culture has a low diagnostic yield, and pleural biopsy, which is the most common way for identification, many times is not readily available for most patients.

Heart and thoracic blood vessel involvement by tuberculosis is a rare disease. Diagnosis of direct cardiac tissue involvement is made in only around 2% of patients [8]. However, pericardial effusions are more common, and tuberculosis can be the culprit of most of the pericardial effusions of patient with a lack of adequate immune system response, reaching almost 70% of them [9]. Aortic tuberculous involvement is also extremely rare and can occur secondary to infection in adjacent tissue and blood dissemination.

Bone and chest wall infection by tuberculosis is also a rare presentation, accounting for approximately 2% of all tuberculosis cases reported [10]. The most common site of musculoskeletal involvement is the spinal bones, but tuberculosis can also invade the ribs, muscles, sternum, and sternoclavicular joints [10]. Most of the infections are also related to adjacent tissue invasion but can also occur secondary to hematogenous and lymphatic dissemination.

4. Tuberculous lymphadenitis

After the mycobacterium is inhaled into the lungs, it is engulfed in macrophages after activation of nonnatural immune system occurs. The immune system forms granulomas that can rupture and infect the adjacent tissue. Mycobacteria can also enter in the lymphatic duct and travel to the lymph node in the proximity. Inside the lymph nodes, the mycobacteria can cause active inflammation and abscesses. Tuberculous lymph node involvement can present as a mass-like lesion but also can cause fissures and ulcers [11]. Thoracic lymphadenitis occurs in the mediastinum and hilar nodes, but lymphadenopathy can also occur in the supraclavicular area and migrate to the neck and face. More common symptoms are those associated to pulmonary tuberculosis but in some patients can present with pain and mass effect. Other patients can present with ulceration of the skin as the nodules progress to an abscess and cause a fistula.

Diagnosis is made by culture and tissue evaluation. Fine needle aspiration is the most common diagnostic evaluation, but other techniques include surgical node excision. Aspiration of the lymph nodes can be done guided by ultrasound or CAT scan. Also, ultrasound- or non-ultrasound-guided bronchoscopic approach can also be done. Fine needle aspiration or direct nodal biopsy has shown similar diagnostic yields in the present literature [1].

Identification of the mycobacteria by acid-fast staining, cultures, and genetic testing has been the principal method of diagnosis. Histologic evidence of granulomatous disease can also help in the diagnosis of negative culture patients in the proper clinical setting.

Treatment for tuberculous lymphadenitis is similar to pulmonary disease: antituberculous antibiotic with isoniazid, rifampin, and ethambutol for 2 months [12], followed by 4–7 months of isoniazid and rifampin. Total duration of disease is about 6–9 months, and length and type of therapy can be affected by other organ involvement, immunosuppressive level of the patient, and culture sensitivities. Surgical and percutaneous drainage can assist in treatment when abscess and fistulas are formed and mass effect is caused by the enlarged nodes.

5. Tuberculous pleurisy

Pleural tissue manifestations of tuberculosis are the second most common finding of thoracic extrapulmonary disease, and it competes with lymphadenitis as the most common extrapulmonary disease presentation. The mycobacteria can reach the pleural cavity by direct parenchymal tissue rupture but also can travel to pleural tissue by the lymphatic system. When the mycobacteria reach the pleural tissue, it can cause a hypersensitivity reaction that produces a lymphocytic inflammatory proliferation that decreases pleural fluid resorption [7]. Also, the inflammatory reaction increases the permeability of the pleural capillaries to proteins and increases the oncotic pressure inside the cavity, increasing the rate of pleural fluid formation [13]. The pleural fluid, rich in cells and protein, obstructs the lymphatic ducts of the parietal pleura and decreases fluid clearance from the pleural space [13]. So, a high rate of fluid formation and the decreased pleural fluid removal lead to the accumulation of pleural fluid and development of pleural effusions. Also, the inflammatory reaction and granuloma formation affect directly the pleural tissue, causing pleural thickening and fibrosis.

Common clinical presentations include symptoms of concomitant pulmonary parenchymal infection as cough, hemoptysis, fever, and weigh loss. Other patients present with pleuritic and nonspecific pain or dyspnea as fluid accumulation causes compression of the lung tissue. Chest wall pain can occur as the parietal pleura is involved and a pleural inflammatory reaction causes abscesses and empyema. The most severe presentation is when the pleural abscess fistulizes to the chest wall, esophagus, main bronchus, and or abdominal cavity, seen as empyema necessitans. Rare cases present without symptoms [14] but have been reported.

Chest images can usually present with a unilateral moderate to large pleural effusion, and almost 90% of patient have concomitant pulmonary parenchymal findings [7]. So, it is always important to rule out active pulmonary disease when pleural tuberculosis is suspected. Nodules, abscesses, and pleural thickening are also common findings on imaging.

Pleural fluid analysis during tuberculous pleurisy shows usually an exudative effusion. As the clinical presentation is usually subacute and chronic inflammation and due to the common immune reaction, the pleural fluid usually presents with lymphocytic cells. Pleural fluid lymphocytic predominance is mostly of more than 50% of the total cell count, and a ratio of lymphocytes to neutrophils is in the range of more than 75% [15]. Cells rarely seen in pleural fluid with tuberculous involvement are mesothelial cells that are present in less than 5% of the total cell count, and eosinophils are rarely in a proportion of more than 10% [7].

Other pleural fluid analyses show increased fluid proteins and low pH and glucose. Lactate dehydrogenase levels are usually high in tuberculous pleurisy, often higher than concomitant blood levels [7].

Pleural fluid stains for tuberculosis as the acid-fast bacillus stains are rarely positive. However, in immunosuppressed patients, for example, HIV positive, it can be positive if it is around 20% of the pleural fluid analysis [16]. Cultures from pleural fluid have slightly higher yield than stains, around 35%, but in concomitant pulmonary tuberculosis, the combination of sputum and pleural fluid culture can have a diagnostic yield of almost 80% [16]. Genetic testing has low sensitivity but good specificity [16], so a positive test is indicative of pleural fluid *Mycobacterium tuberculosis* presence, but a negative test does not rule out the pleural involvement.

Adenosine deaminase (ADA) is a lymphocyte-produced enzyme for metabolism of the components of the DNA. ADA helps during T-cell differentiation and proliferation, and knowing the usual immune reaction activated by the tuberculous bacilli, it is expected that ADA would be high during pleural tissue involvement. Levels of this enzyme have been available during years, and its use has been extensively discussed. In high prevalent populations, a high level is almost diagnostic despite negative cultures of the mycobacterium [17]. The contrary is also considered correct: pleural cavity involvement can be ruled out when a patient in low-prevalence population has low levels of ADA in the pleural fluid. Suggested cutoff values for diagnosis for highly suggested disease are 65–70 IU/L. Levels of less than 35 IU/L have a high negative predictive value for disease in low-incidence populations [17].

Other tests that can be done for identification of tuberculous pleural effusion include genetic testing with polymerase chain reaction, measurement of γ-interferon levels, and interferon release assays. However, those tests have not been readily available and standardized for general use.

Pleural biopsy has the highest diagnostic yield until this time. Biopsy can be done using blind or image-guided percutaneous needle pleural cut. Images used to guide biopsy include ultrasound and CAT scan. Thoracoscopic and surgical pleural biopsy are more invasive alternatives. Tissue evaluation of the parietal pleural tissue can show caseous granuloma and the presence of acid-fast bacilli. Cultures of the pleural tissue have shown the highest yield (75–90%), increasing the diagnosis rate when the biopsy is guided by images [15].

The most efficient way of establishing a diagnosis for pleural tuberculous involvement is throughout a compressive and progressive evaluation. First, ruling out pulmonary parenchymal involvement should be done. Evaluation of the sputum for acid-fast bacilli and cultures is the first step. If pulmonary involvement is ruled out, in the presence of a lymphocytic predominant pleural effusion, pretest probability of pleural tuberculous infection must be taken into account. In low-prevalence populations, a low ADA (less than 35 IU/L) almost rules out the disease. In high-prevalence populations, a high ADA (more than 65 IU/L) is highly suggestive of pleural disease, and treatment can be considered. In a patient with ADA levels in between 35 and 65 IU/L, pleural biopsy can be done, and if typical granulomas are seen, therapy can be considered even with negative cultures. A positive culture would warrant an antibiotic therapy.

Therapy for tuberculous pleural involvement often is similar to pulmonary active infection, as it usually presents with concomitant disease. Usually it includes isoniazid, rifampin, ethambutol, and pyrazinamide for the first 8 weeks or until sensitivities are obtained, and then 16 weeks of isoniazid and rifampin are completed to a total of 6 months. Direct observe therapy is recommended during the completion of treatment [7].

Adding systemic steroids for pleural tuberculosis is not recommended as no benefit has been seen [18], and usually complications of immunosuppressive therapy add morbidity and mortality to the patients. In some patients with persistent pain and fever symptoms, systemic steroids can be considered [7] for a short period of time, until symptoms subside. Surgical evacuation with simultaneous antituberculosis antibiotics is the treatment option for empyema. It usually requires complex decortication and debridement of tissue and abscess area, with reconstruction of the surrounding tissue as in the case of empyema necessitans.

6. Cardiac and pericardial disease

Tuberculous involvement of the heart can include infection of the pericardium (most common), the cardiac muscle, and the large blood vessels as the aorta.

Pericardial involvement is similar to pleural tuberculosis. The pericardium acquires the infection by lymphatic or hematogenous spread of the bacteria, as well as rupture of granulomas on an adjacent tissue. Once the mycobacteria reach the tissue, it causes similar hypersensitive reaction inside the pericardium leaded by T cells. This inflammatory process induces a granulomatous reaction that progresses to a fibrinous and serosanguineous effusion and produces pericardial thickening and fibrosis [18]. Impaired lymphatic drainage can worsen the process and cause rapid accumulation of fluid.

Clinical presentations can vary from systemic symptoms due to pulmonary and other organ infection to chest pain and congestive heart failure. Rapid fluid accumulation can cause vascular collapse due to cardiac tamponade. Asymptomatic pericardial effusion is very uncommon.

Diagnosis of pericardial involvement is made by similar mechanisms as pleural disease. Analysis of pleural fluid aspirated using direct visualization with ultrasound or CAT scan can be done. Also, surgical exploration is an alternative when those methods are not available, and other diseases are also considered. Pericardial fluid analysis findings are similar to tuberculous pleural fluid, including lymphocytic cellular predominance, low glucose and pH, high LDH levels, and similar levels of ADA. Biopsies usually show granulomas and AFB, and culture for mycobacteria can be positive. Empiric treatment response can be highly suggestive of diagnosis in high-risk populations with no conclusive diagnosis, but confirmation of infection is the recommended evaluation.

Other cardiac involvement presentation is direct invasion of the myocardial tissue and endocarditis. This is a very rare presentation and is usually fatal. Clinical findings include symptoms similar to a cardiomyopathy with heart failure, arrhythmias, conduction blocks, cardiac output blocks, valvulopathy, and aneurysms [8]. Diagnosis is usually done with an autopsy due to the severity of the cases.

The aorta can also be involved after hematogenous involvement or due to proximity in concomitant cardiac disease. In nonfatal cases, diagnosis is done after reviewing tissue from repaired aneurysms [19].

Therapy for cardiac tuberculosis includes drainage of pericardial effusions, by surgical or percutaneous methods, with simultaneous antituberculous antibiotics for 6–9 months. Systemic steroids during pericardial effusion have not demonstrated less progression to fibrosis in the pericardium or less requirement of surgical interventions, but some studies suggest a decrease in mortality [20]. Antituberculous therapy has an initial regime of four drugs (isoniazid, rifampin, ethambutol, and pyrazinamide) and then two drugs, as sensitivities become available. Surgical interventions are indicated in some cases of valvular or large vessel involvement.

7. Bone and musculoskeletal involvement

The most common presentation of musculoskeletal involvement is vertebral and chest wall invasion secondary to hematogenous, lymphatic, and adjacent tissue infection spreading. When the spine is involved, it is known as Pott's disease. The name originated from the description of tuberculous infection of the spine by Sir Percivall Pott, a British surgeon, in 1779 [21]. The tuberculous bacilli invade the bone and vertebral disk with an inflammatory and mass-like process that destroys the tissue causing fractures and can progress to cord compression.

Clinical presentation will vary according to deepness of tissue invasion and localization. Images usually show the lesions and guide the tissue diagnosis. Confirmation of tuberculosis involvement is done by tissue diagnosis and cultures. The treatment includes a similar antituberculous drug regime to other sites and surgery to correct possible mechanical damage.

8. Conclusion

Thoracic extrapulmonary tuberculosis is a disease characterized for *Mycobacterium tuberculosis* involvement outside the pulmonary parenchyma and inside the chest cavity. It has a variety of presentations according the tissue affected. More common presentations include the lymph nodes and pleural tissue, but rare cases present with myocardial and chest wall invasion. Cases can be fatal. Therapy usually is mainly based on antituberculous therapy, but some patients require percutaneous and surgical procedures. Clinical suspicion and the correct work-up usually led to the diagnosis.

Author details

Onix J. Cantres-Fonseca
Department of Pulmonary & Critical Care Medicine & Internal Medicine, VA Caribbean Heath System, San Juan, Puerto Rico

*Address all correspondence to: onixcantres@gmail.com

References

[1] Salvador F et al. Epidemiology and diagnosis of tuberculous lymphadenitis in a tuberculosis low-burden country. Medicine (Baltimore). 2015;**94**(4):509

[2] Ravimohan S et al. Tuberculosis and lung damage: From epidemiology to pathophysiology. European Respiratory Review. 2018;**27**:170077

[3] Cantres O et al. Extra pulmonary tuberculosis: An overview. In: Role of Microbes in Human Health and Diseases. London: IntechOpen; 2018

[4] Mazza-Stadler J, Nicod L. Extra pulmonary tuberculosis. Revue des Maladies Respiratoires. 2012;**29**(4):566-578

[5] Kulchavenya E. Extrapulmonary tuberculosis: Are statistical reports accurate? Therapeutic Advances in Infectious Disease. 2014;**2**(2):61-70

[6] García-Rodríguez JF, Álvarez-Díaz H, Lorenzo-García M, Mariño Callejo A, Fernández-Rial A, Sesma-Sánchez P. Extrapulmonary tuberculosis: Epidemiology and risk factors. Enfermedades Infecciosas y Microbiología Clínica. 2011;**29**(7):502-509

[7] Cohen L et al. Tuberculous pleural effusion. Turkish Thoracic Journal. 2015;**16**(1):1-9

[8] Agarwal R et al. Tuberculous dilated cardiomyopathy: An under-recognized entity? BMC Infectious Diseases. 2005;**5**:29

[9] Reuter H et al. Epidemiology of pericardial effusions at a large academic hospital in South Africa. Epidemiology and Infection. 2005;**133**(3):393-399

[10] Grover SB et al. Chest wall tuberculosis–A clinical and imaging experience. Indian Journal of Radiology and Imaging. 2011;**21**(1):28-33

[11] Hedge S et al. Tuberculous lymphadenitis: Early diagnosis and intervention. Journal of International Oral Health. 2014;**6**(6):96-98

[12] Cambelle IA. Tubercle. 1990;**71**(1):1-3

[13] Light R. Update on tuberculous pleural effusion. Respirology. 2010

[14] Shinohara T et al. Asymptomatic primary tuberculous pleurisy with intense 18-fluorodeoxyglucose uptake mimicking malignant mesothelioma. BMC Infectious Diseases. 2013;**13**:12

[15] Shaw J et al. Pleural tuberculosis: a concise clinical review. The Clinical Respiratory Journal. 2018:1779

[16] Zhai K et al. Tuberculous pleural effusion. Journal of Thoracic Disease. 2016 Jul;**8**(7):E486-E494

[17] Aggarwal A et al. Adenosine deaminase for diagnosis of tuberculous pleural effusion: A systematic review and meta-analysis. PLoS One. 2019;**14**(3):e0213728

[18] Galarza I et al. Randomised trial of corticosteroids in the treatment of tuberculous pleurisy. Thorax. 1995;**50**(12):1305-1307

[19] Pathirana U et al. Ascending aortic aneurysm caused by *Mycobacterium tuberculosis*. BMC Research Notes. 2015;**8**:659

[20] Mayosi B et al. Tuberculous pericarditis. Circulation. 2005;**112**:3608-3616

[21] Garg RK et al. Spinal tuberculosis: A review. The Journal of Spinal Cord Medicine. 2011;**34**(5):440-454

Section 3

Cor Pulmonale and Ultrasound

Chapter 6

Application of Thoracic Ultrasonography for Acute Cor Pulmonale in Acute Respiratory Distress Syndrome Patients

You Shang and Ting Zhou

Abstract

Beneficial therapeutic interventions for acute respiratory distress syndrome (ARDS) include lung protective ventilation; however, ventilator may cause or sometimes worsen acute cor pulmonale (ACP) induced by pulmonary gas exchange disorder and pulmonary vascular dysfunction due to ARDS. The incidence of ACP was 22–50% in mechanically ventilated patients. Currently, point-of-care ultrasound has been widely used in ARDS patients, which becomes much more important in the early detection and management of ARDS and its complications. Application of lung ultrasound combined with echocardiography could monitor respiratory status, hemodynamics, and cardiac function and optimize the ventilation setting in order to protect both lung and right ventricle. This chapter will discuss the pathophysiology of ACP associated with ARDS and the use of point-of-care ultrasound to make protective strategies for lung and right ventricle in detail.

Keywords: acute respiratory distress syndrome, acute cor pulmonale, point-of-care ultrasound, organ protection

1. Introduction

The concept of acute respiratory distress syndrome (ARDS) was first described about five decades ago [1], which is characterized by the acute development of hypoxemia accompanied with bilateral lung infiltrates [2]. ARDS is responsible not only for infections, shock, and multiple organ dysfunction syndromes but also for acute cor pulmonale (ACP) and right ventricular failure in critical ill patients. The mortality of ARDS is 40% approximately in intensive care unit [3], and almost 25% of mechanically ventilated patients could be affected by ARDS [4]. Lung protective mechanical ventilation using low tidal volume and high positive end expiratory pressure (PEEP) and other therapeutic interventions such as fluid restrictive, prone position, neuromuscular blockade, lung recruitment, and sometimes venovenous extracorporeal membrane oxygenation (VV ECMO) for severe cases may be beneficial [5–9]; however, none of them are promising and may cause other complications, for instance, low tidal volume and high PEEP may lead to hypercapnia and consecutive right heart failure [4].

In 1977, it was first found that some ARDS patients accompanied with deleterious effect on pulmonary system and increased pulmonary vascular resistance, or even pulmonary hypertension [10]. Until 2001, it was reported that there was 25% ARDS patients occurring acute cor pulmonale (ACP) when they were receiving lung protective mechanical ventilation with low tidal volume and high positive end expiratory pressure (PEEP) [11]. The incidence of ACP was much higher in severe ARDS patients whose PaO_2/FiO_2 were lower than 100 mmHg. The morbidity was over 50% [12]. In terms of mortality, it was over 60% in moderate to severe ARDS patients (Berlin definition) with ACP, which was defined by transesophageal ultrasound (TEE); however, the incidence was 30% if without ACP [13]. We will discuss it in detail in this chapter.

2. Pathophysiology of acute cor pulmonale (ACP) in ARDS patients

The main function of right heart is maintaining adequate pulmonary perfusion pressure to deliver desaturated mixed venous blood to the respiratory membrane and low systemic venous pressure to prevent organ congestion. The right ventricle is sensitive to changes in afterload because it is anatomically adapted for the generation of low-pressure perfusion [4, 14–16].

Hypoxia induced by ARDS will cause the construction of pulmonary vessels. Pulmonary vasoconstriction could be caused not only by hypoxia but also by damaged pulmonary capillary coagulation, which may result in microvascular obstruction in the lung. In early phase of ARDS, microvascular thrombi could be seen in the histological studies. Those obstructed capillaries could lose their vascular structures in late phase of ARDS [17]. Lung protective mechanical ventilation with low tidal volume may also lead to hypercapnia in ARDS patients, aggravate the constriction of pulmonary arteries, and increase the pulmonary vascular resistance [18]. Furthermore, microvascular obstruction damaged coagulation and inflammation in ARDS contributes to increased afterload of right ventricle and induces right heart failure [19]. When right heart fails to deliver adequate volume to pulmonary circulation, the left heart will be affected with low cardiac output, decreased systemic hypotension, and multiple organ malperfusion.

Mechanical ventilation is also an important determinant to ACP and right ventricular failure; however, there is no robust evidence to support a definitive causal relationship between ACP and respiratory mechanics parameters, such as plateaus pressure, driving pressure, PEEP, and so on. If Vt or PEEP is inappropriate high, pleural pressure will increase and affect venous return of right atrium [20]. Even 6 ml/kg Vt still caused lung overdistension in one-third of ARDS patient [21]. Too low PEEP also results in atelectasis and progressive lung injury [22]. Function of right heart relies on the intrapleural pressure, gas exchange, and balance of lung recruitment and overdistension [13]. A large prospective observational clinical study had been designed to find that there are three physiological and one clinical parameters that could reflect the risk of ACP and would facilitate the attending physician in selecting patients who require echocardiographic assessment and close monitoring. The four variables were as follows: (1) pneumonia as a cause of ARDS; (2) driving pressure (plateau pressure-total positive end-expiratory pressure) >18 cm H_2O; (3) $PaO_2/FiO_2 < 150$ mmHg; and (4) $PaCO_2 > 48$ mmHg. One score for each variable. Patients with a score higher than two had a higher risk of ACP (19, 34, and 74% for risk scores of 2, 3, and 4, respectively) [16].

Damage to either gas exchange or respiratory mechanics may excessive increases preload or afterload of right ventricle, or injury that results in decreased right ventricular contractility [4]. However, due to anatomic structure of right ventricle, the tolerance of acute increases of afterload is poor, and right heart undergoes dilate to afford it (according to Starling's law). Then, the decrease in right ventricular ejection is responsible for a decrease in left ventricular preload, and right ventricular dilatation is also responsible for left ventricular compression by a septal shift because of the inextensible pericardium [11, 23]. So, decreased left ventricular ejection lowers the cardiac output, systemic blood pressure, and then the coronary artery flow. Decreased coronary artery flow aggravates hypoxia of myocardium; meanwhile, the oxygen consumption of myocardium is increased. When there is an imbalance of oxygen demand and supply, the vicious cycle begins; the more the right heart dilates, the less the right heart coronary blood flow, and the reduced right heart function [4, 24].

In ARDS patients, we try to achieve a balance between maintaining lung open and adequate right heart function; thus, we need to ultrasound to assist us to monitor both lung and heart function at meantime [3].

3. Monitor pulmonary function using point-of-care ultrasound in clinical setting

Point-of-care ultrasound is a readily, minimal invasive, no-radiation and repeatable bedside tool in clinical settings, which has increased widely over the past decade in the intensive care units and plays a very important role in helping intensivists' diagnosing and treating critical ill patients [25].

Point-of-care pulmonary ultrasound scan could be used to assist the diagnosis in the early phase of ARDS. Suspected ARDS could be confirmed by pulmonary ultrasonography scan through the following typical patterns characterized by B-lines, spared areas, pleural line thickening, and subpleural consolidations [26]. The blue protocol indicates the number and thickness of B-lines permitting a semiquantitative evaluation of the amount of extravascular lung water and lung density as well. Lung ultrasound could determine the consolidation of local lung segment, usually in the basal and posterior area, showing hepatization (tissue pattern) in the presence of air bronchograms in 83.3% ARDS patients [27, 28]. Lung ultrasound could also assist intensivists to evaluate proper PEEP in lung recruitment in ARDS patient, avoiding high PEEP induced lung injury. When localized the consolidation of lung segments with lung ultrasound with real-time monitoring, increasing PEEP stepwisely could reduce the degree of nonaerated lung area, while no hemodynamic deterioration was noted [29]. Although CT is considered a valid technique to estimate lung recruitment in ARDS patients by quantifying the amount of tissue according to the different lung recruitment maneuvers, lung ultrasound provides higher safety and available at bedsides and allows continuous monitoring of the nonaerated dependent lung regions, avoiding derecruitment in clinical practice [30, 31].

4. Critical care echocardiography

Ultrasound has been applied in critical ill patients worldwide, which guided the intensivists establish not only all sorts of catheters, like central veins and arteries, but also thoracentesis, peritoneocentesis, and sometimes rachiocentesis. In the other words, ultrasound provides a real-time view and assists the preformation of intensivists under any critical situations. Despite its easily application and availability in any situation, ultrasound has become much more important in management of ARDS patients when evaluating their cardiac function because those patients had complex interactions among the lung, the ventilation, and the right ventricle [32]. Recently, there were debates about the choice of the modality of echocardiography, either transthoracic (TTE), or transesophageal (TEE). Most documents indicated that TEE is superior to TTE for diagnosis of ACP or right ventricular dysfunction in mechanically ventilated patient with moderate to severe ARDS, as it overcomes technical problems associated with acoustic views and measurements that can usually be performed easily [32, 33]. Another advantage about TEE is providing safely and efficiently when ARDS patients need long duration of prone position or have excessive pneumoderma affecting the ultrasound images [34]. Furthermore, some articles also indicated that TEE has high accuracy than TTE in observing ACP if the patient was mechanical ventilated with high PEEP [33, 35]. Compared to TEE, the sensitivity of TTE for diagnosis of right ventricular dysfunction was only 60% (95% CI, 41–77%) [36]. However, if both TEE and TTE could be chosen in the ICU, the intensivists should consider individual clinical conditions of the patients, experience of using echocardiography, and the clinical settings of the ward. The related invasiveness of TEE should be considered too [37].

As mentioned above, the definition of ACP is acute increased right ventricular afterload, which resulted in right ventricular dilatation and may compromise left ventricular filling. Right ventricular volume overload is defined as dilatation of the right ventricle that could be easily observed with echocardiography, while right ventricular pressure overload is defined as dyskinetic movement of the septum during end-systole. Right ventricular volume and right ventricular pressure could interact with each other [37, 38].

There are many echocardiographic manifestations of ACP. Echocardiography of ACP in an ARDS patient ventilated with a lung protective approach is characterized by (A) a severe dilatation of the right ventricle, a mark, or of right ventricular failure and (B) a paradoxical septal motion with the "D-shape" of the left ventricle, reflecting that right ventricular failure is related to systolic overload (abrupt increase in right ventricular afterload) [32].

Based on the visual image of the right heart provided by two-dimensional echocardiography, assessment of right ventricular size is a widely adopted method, by comparing the right ventricular end-diastolic area (RVEDA) with the left ventricular end-diastolic area (LVEDA) [24, 32, 39]. The RVEDA/LVEDA ratio between 0.6 and 1 indicates moderate ACP, while the RVEDA/LVEDA ratio greater than 1 indicates severe ACP. ACP diagnosis by echocardiographic has been defined as the combination of an RVEDA/LVEDA ratio > 0.6 and the presence of paradoxical septal motion during end-systole on parasternal short axis and apical four-chamber views, which now considered to be gold standard [4, 24, 33].

The statement from the Heart Failure Association and the Working Group on Pulmonary Circulation and Right Ventricular Function of the European Society of Cardiology indicated 12 echocardiographic parameters in the assessment of right ventricular failure, which were (A) pericardial fluid >5 mm in diastole; (B) RV wall thickness > 5 mm; (C) inferior vena cava diameter > 21 mm, inspiration collapse <50% suggests high RA pressure; (D) tricuspid regurgitation peak systolic velocity of TR > 2.8 m/s; (E) tricuspid annular plane systolic excursion TAPSE < 17 mm; (F) right ventricle dilation RVEDD/LVEDD > 1.0, right ventricle basal diameter > 41 mm; (G) right ventricle fractional area change, FAC < 35%; (H) ventricular interdependence: septal shift, D-shaped left ventricle; (I) systolic S′ velocity of tricuspid annulus < 9.5 cm/s by Doppler Tissue Imaging; (J) longitudinal strain of right ventricle free wall < 20%; (K) right ventricular index of myocardial performance, RIMP > 0.54 by Doppler Tissue Imaging; and (L) 3D right ventricular ejection fraction < 45% [40].

5. Right heart protection

Effective treatment of acute cor pulmonale or right heart failure requires an experienced and skilled ICU team to rapidly assess and treat. Lung protective mechanical ventilated strategy could not guarantee to protect the function of right heart for the intensivists. Performing bedside echocardiography could help in tailoring the ventilator management to decrease right ventricular afterload when ACP is detected, thus potentially avoiding further deterioration toward severe ACP [16, 41]. Moreover, within the visual image of the right heart provided by two-dimensional echocardiography, early observation of right ventricular dysfunction using echocardiography could help the intensivists to differentiate the pathophysiology of ACP and make appropriated treatments to optimizing right ventricular preload, increasing right ventricular contractility, and reducing right ventricular afterload, such as therapeutic treatment or prone position [12, 42]. Furthermore, echocardiography could also provide a continuous visual image after the treatments and help to evaluate whether the heart function is improved or not. In other words, with echocardiography, the morbidity and mortality of ACP in ARDS patient might be reduced, and there is a huge need to design more clinical trials using echocardiography in critical ill patients with ARDS.

6. Conclusion

Because of the coupling between lung and heart, the right ventricle is also involved in ARDS either primarily or by the application of mechanical ventilation. Acute cor pulmonale is seen with increasing frequency in the intensive care unit. The incidence of acute cor pulmonale during ARDS is, even if under protective ventilation, not negligible. The use of echocardiography combined with lung ultrasound is important for early detection of acute cor pulmonale and identification of the appropriate ventilator strategy to preserve heart-to-lung interaction. Furthermore, right now, there is no clinical practice guideline or therapeutic intervention focus on the right ventricular protective ventilation strategy in ARDS patients with high risk of ACP. More research should be done to establish how to differentiate patients with high risk of ACP, immediate assessment by echocardiography, and early interventions.

Author details

You Shang* and Ting Zhou
Department of Critical Care Medicine, Union Hospital, Tongji Medical College, Huazhong University of Science and Technology, Wuhan, China.

*Address all correspondence to: you_shang@yahoo.com

References

[1] Ashbaugh DG, Bigelow DB, Petty TL, Levine BE. Acute respiratory distress in adults. Lancet. 1967;**2**(7511):319-323. DOI: 10.1016/s0140-6736(67)90168-7

[2] Ranieri VM, Rubenfeld GD, Thompson BT, et al. Acute respiratory distress syndrome: The Berlin Definition. JAMA. 2012;307;(23):2526-2533. DOI: 10.1001/jama.2012.5669, 10.1001/jama.2012.5669

[3] Zochios V, Parhar K, Tunnicliffe W. The right ventricle in ARDS. Chest. 2017;**152**(1):181-193. DOI: 10.1016/j.chest.2017.02.019

[4] Mathieu G, Antoine VB. Hemodynamic monitoring of ARDS by critical care echocardiography. J Emerg Crit Care Med. 2019;**3**:36. DOI: 10.21037/jeccm.2019.07.04

[5] Brower RG, Matthay MA, Morris A, et al. Ventilation with lower tidal volumes as compared with traditional tidal volumes for acute lung injury and the acute respiratory distress syndrome. The New England Journal of Medicine. 2000;**342**(18):1301-1308. DOI: 10.1056/NEJM200005043421801

[6] Guérin C, Reignier J, Richard JC, et al. Prone positioning in severe acute respiratory distress syndrome. The New England Journal of Medicine. 2013;**368**(23):2159-2168. DOI: 10.1056/NEJMoa1214103

[7] Wiedemann HP, Wheeler AP, Bernard GR, et al. Comparison of two fluid-management strategies in acute lung injury. The New England Journal of Medicine. 2006;**354**(24):2564-2575. DOI: 10.1056/NEJMoa062200

[8] Papazian L, Forel JM, Gacouin A, et al. Neuromuscular blockers in early acute respiratory distress syndrome. The New England Journal of Medicine. 2010;**363**(12):1107-1116. DOI: 10.1056/NEJMoa1005372

[9] Bunge JJH, Caliskan K, Gommers D, Reis MD. Right ventricular dysfunction during acute respiratory distress syndrome and veno-venous extracorporeal membrane oxygenation. J Thorac Dis. 2018;**10**(Suppl 5): S674-S682. DOI: 10.21037/jtd.2017.10.75

[10] Zapol WM, Snider MT. Pulmonary hypertension in severe acute respiratory failure. The New England Journal of Medicine. 1977;**296**(9):476-480. DOI: 10.1056/NEJM197703032960903

[11] Vieillard-Baron A, Schmitt JM, Augarde R, et al. Acute cor pulmonale in acute respiratory distress syndrome submitted to protective ventilation: Incidence, clinical implications, and prognosis. Critical Care Medicine. 2001;**29**(8):1551-1555. DOI: 10.1097/00003246-200108000-00009

[12] Vieillard-Baron A, Charron C, Caille V, et al. Prone positioning unloads the right ventricle in severe ARDS. Chest. 2007;**132**(5):1440-1446. DOI: 10.1378/chest.07-1013

[13] Boissier F, Katsahian S, Razazi K, et al. Prevalence and prognosis of cor pulmonale during protective ventilation for acute respiratory distress syndrome. Intensive Care Medicine. 2013;**39**(10):1725-1733. DOI: 10.1007/s00134-013-2941-9

[14] Greyson CR. Pathophysiology of right ventricular failure. Critical Care Medicine. 2008;**36**(1 Suppl): S57-S65. DOI: 10.1097/01.CCM.0000296265.52518.70

[15] Zochios V, Jones N. Acute right heart syndrome in the critically ill patient. Heart Lung Vessel. 2014;**6**(3):157-170

[16] Mekontso Dessap A, Boissier F, Charron C, et al. Acute cor pulmonale during protective ventilation for acute respiratory distress syndrome: Prevalence, predictors, and clinical impact. Intensive Care Medicine. 2016;**42**(5):862-870. DOI: 10.1007/s00134-015-4141-2

[17] Bellingan GJ. The pulmonary physician in critical care * 6: The pathogenesis of ALI/ARDS. Thorax. 2002;**57**(6):540-546. DOI: 10.1136/thorax.57.6.540

[18] Mekontso Dessap A, Charron C, Devaquet J, et al. Impact of acute hypercapnia and augmented positive end-expiratory pressure on right ventricle function in severe acute respiratory distress syndrome. Intensive Care Medicine. 2009;**35**(11):1850-1858. DOI: 10.1007/s00134-009-1569-2

[19] Jardin F, Vieillard-Baron A. Is there a safe plateau pressure in ARDS? The right heart only knows. Intensive Care Medicine. 2007;**33**(3):444-447. DOI: 10.1007/s00134-007-0552-z

[20] Lansdorp B, Hofhuizen C, van Lavieren M, et al. Mechanical ventilation-induced intrathoracic pressure distribution and heart-lung interactions*. Critical Care Medicine. 2014;**42**(9):1983-1990. DOI: 10.1097/CCM.0000000000000345

[21] Reis Miranda D, Klompe L, Mekel J, et al. Open lung ventilation does not increase right ventricular outflow impedance: An echo-Doppler study. Critical Care Medicine. 2006;**34**(10):2555-2560. DOI: 10.1097/01.CCM.0000239118.05093.EE

[22] Duggan M, McCaul CL, McNamara PJ, et al. Atelectasis causes vascular leak and lethal right ventricular failure in uninjured rat lungs. American Journal of Respiratory and Critical Care Medicine. 2003;**167**(12):1633-1640. DOI: 10.1164/rccm.200210-1215OC

[23] Repessé X, Charron C, Vieillard-Baron A. Acute respiratory distress syndrome: The heart side of the moon. Current Opinion in Critical Care. 2016;**22**(1):38-44. DOI: 10.1097/MCC.0000000000000267

[24] Jones N, Burns AT, Prior DL. Echocardiographic assessment of the right ventricle-state of the art. Heart, Lung & Circulation. 2019;**28**(9):1339-1350. DOI: 10.1016/j.hlc.2019.04.016

[25] Corradi F, Brusasco C, Pelosi P. Chest ultrasound in acute respiratory distress syndrome. Current Opinion in Critical Care. 2014;**20**(1):98-103. DOI: 10.1097/MCC.0000000000000042

[26] Lichtenstein DA, Mezière GA. The BLUE-points: Three standardized points used in the BLUE-protocol for ultrasound assessment of the lung in acute respiratory failure. Critical Ultrasound Journal. 2011;**3**(2):109-110. DOI: 10.1007/s13089-011-0066-3

[27] Lichtenstein DA. Lung ultrasound in the critically ill. Clinical Intensive Care. 2005;**16**:79-87. DOI: 10.1080/09563070500131027

[28] Copetti R, Soldati G, Copetti P. Chest sonography: A useful tool to differentiate acute cardiogenic pulmonary edema from acute respiratory distress syndrome. Cardiovascular Ultrasound. 2008;**6**:16. DOI: 10.1186/1476-7120-6-16

[29] Stefanidis K, Dimopoulos S, Tripodaki ES, et al. Lung sonography and recruitment in patients with early acute respiratory distress syndrome: A pilot study. Critical Care. 2011;**15**(4):R185. DOI: 10.1186/cc10338

[30] Bouhemad B, Brisson H, Le-Guen M, et al. Bedside ultrasound assessment of positive end-expiratory pressure-induced lung recruitment. American Journal of Respiratory and Critical Care Medicine.

2011;**183**(3):341-347. DOI: 10.1164/rccm.201003-0369OC

[31] Via G, Lichtenstein D, Mojoli F, et al. Whole lung lavage: A unique model for ultrasound assessment of lung aeration changes. Intensive Care Medicine. 2010;**36**(6):999-1007. DOI: 10.1007/s00134-010-1834-4

[32] Vieillard-Baron A, Prin S, Chergui K, et al. Echo-Doppler demonstration of acute cor pulmonale at the bedside in the medical intensive care unit. American Journal of Respiratory and Critical Care Medicine. 2002;**166**(10):1310-1319. DOI: 10.1164/rccm.200202-146CC

[33] Lhéritier G, Legras A, Caille A, et al. Prevalence and prognostic value of acute cor pulmonale and patent foramen ovale in ventilated patients with early acute respiratory distress syndrome: A multicenter study. Intensive Care Med. 2013;**39**(10):1734-1742. DOI: 10.1007/s00134-013-3017-6

[34] Mekontso Dessap A, Proost O, Boissier F, et al. Transesophageal echocardiography in prone position during severe acute respiratory distress syndrome. Intensive Care Medicine. 2011;**37**(3):430-434. DOI: 10.1007/s00134-010-2114-z

[35] Cook CH, Praba AC, Beery PR, Martin LC. Transthoracic echocardiography is not cost-effective in critically ill surgical patients. The Journal of Trauma. 2002;**52**(2):280-284. DOI: 10.1097/00005373-200202000-00013

[36] Fichet J, Moreau L, Genée O, et al. Feasibility of right ventricular longitudinal systolic function evaluation with transthoracic echocardiographic indices derived from tricuspid annular motion: A preliminary study in acute respiratory distress syndrome. Echocardiography. 2012;**29**(5):513-521. DOI: 10.1111/j.1540-8175.2011.01650.x

[37] Stanko LK, Jacobsohn E, Tam JW, et al. Transthoracic echocardiography: Impact on diagnosis and management in tertiary care intensive care units. Anaesthesia and Intensive Care. 2005;**33**(4):492-496. DOI: 10.1177/0310057X0503300411

[38] Ryan T, Petrovic O, Dillon JC, et al. An echocardiographic index for separation of right ventricular volume and pressure overload. Journal of the American College of Cardiology. 1985;**5**(4):918-927. DOI: 10.1016/s0735-1097(85)80433-2

[39] Frémont B, Pacouret G, Jacobi D, et al. Prognostic value of echocardiographic right/left ventricular end-diastolic diameter ratio in patients with acute pulmonary embolism: Results from a monocenter registry of 1,416 patients. Chest. 2008;**133**(2):358-362. DOI: 10.1378/chest.07-1231

[40] Harjola VP, Mebazaa A, Čelutkienė J, et al. Contemporary management of acute right ventricular failure: A statement from the heart failure association and the working group on pulmonary circulation and right ventricular function of the European Society of Cardiology. European Journal of Heart Failure. 2016;**18**(3):226-241. DOI: 10.1002/ejhf.478

[41] Vieillard-Baron A, Price LC, Matthay MA. Acute cor pulmonale in ARDS. Intensive Care Medicine. 2013;**39**(10):1836-1838. DOI: 10.1007/s00134-013-3045-2

[42] Galiatsou E, Kostanti E, Svarna E, et al. Prone position augments recruitment and prevents alveolar overinflation in acute lung injury. American Journal of Respiratory and Critical Care Medicine. 2006;**174**(2):187-197. DOI: 10.1164/rccm.200506-899OC

Section 4

Rehabilitation

Chapter 7

Long-Term Adherence and Maintenance of Benefits in Pulmonary Rehabilitation

Hulya Sahin

Abstract

Pulmonary rehabilitation (PR) is a comprehensive intervention in chronic lung diseases, including personalized special therapies, exercise training, education and behavioral changes to improve the physical and psychological status of the patients, and aims to promote behavior that helps improve health status in the long term. A personalized PR program administered by a multidisciplinary team is recently considered a standard and complementary treatment method in chronic lung diseases. After the PR program, dyspnea of COPD patients decreases and their exercise capacities increase. Their daily life activities and physical activities increase. Their functional dependence decreases and quality of life increases. It presents a perfect opportunity to provide self-management and independence for the patients and improve their quality of life. Studies have shown that, unless there is a structured maintenance program, after an average of 6–12 months following PR programs, the gains that are realized start to decrease. Decrease of gains due to causes like a decrease in compliance to exercises, disease progress, attacks and co-morbidities. Causes such as decreased compliance to exercise, progression of the disease, attacks and comorbidities play a role in reducing gains. Especially in advanced age and in the presence of severe disease, the gain in exercise tolerance is lost more rapidly. The methods used and the results obtained to ensure the continuation of the gains differ.

Keywords: pulmonary rehabilitation, maintenance, adherence, chronic respiratory disease, COPD

1. Introduction

Based on hard evidence, pulmonary rehabilitation (PR) increases exercise capacity, decreases perception of dyspnea and improves the quality of life [1, 2]. Therefore, it has become a standard treatment in the management of patients suffering from chronic respiratory disease [1]. The basic component of this comprehensive program is exercise training and it is intended to break the vicious circle of dyspnea and deconditioning [3, 4]. Maintenance of the benefits in patients who participated a PR program depends on increasing the physical activity and changing the lifestyle. A successful PR program requires the patients to make a series of complicated changes in their behaviors such as regularly exercising, adaptation to treatment, learning the methods of breathing and changing lifestyle [5].

In terms of maintaining the benefits, patient's failure to do physical activities and change the lifestyle after PR constitutes the major problem [6]. According to In a study which assessed the COPD patients 3 times within 1 year after PR, it was found that the daily step count, time spent for sedentary activities and daily physical activities did not change [4]. Likewise, when COPD patients administered PR were assessed 3 and 6 months after the program, it was seen that the time allocated for walking had not changed. In COPD patients, increased physical activity after PR depends on two factors: frequency of supervised exercise and the duration of the program [6]. While offering education three times weekly ensures an increase in the physical activity, providing education for two times is insufficient [7]. While a 3-month exercise program had no effect, 6-month supervised exercise program increased physical activity [8].

2. Maintenance of benefits in pulmonary rehabilitation

The benefits start to diminish over 6–12 months in the absence of structured maintenance programs after the program [6, 9]. Reasons such as decreased adherence to exercise, progression of the disease and attacks are responsible for this decrease [9]. The benefit in exercise tolerance diminishes more rapidly especially in old age and in the presence of severe disease [3]. To maintain the benefits, repeating the program once a year or in cases where there is a decrease in exercise capacity, worsening in quality of life or increase in symptoms may be used a method [1]. A part of the COPD patients who accomplished the PR program were administered repeat PR program and the walk distance was observed to increase similar to the first program. It was determined that the maximum decrease in walk distance occurred when there is a 25-month period between two programs, and therefore, it was stated that the repeat program should be started before 25 months [1]. In COPD patients attended to PR program for two consecutive years were observed to lose the benefits in exercise tolerance and perception of dyspnea 1 year later, however they maintained the improvement in quality of life. In the meantime, annual number of bed-days and attacks decreased more. This study indicated that the repeated PR ensures maintaining the quality of life as well as decrease in number of attacks and hospitalization although the benefits in exercise capacity and perception of dyspnea were not maintained [10]. In COPD patients who attended a PR program for three consecutive years, the decrease in FEV1 was observed to be less compared to those who did not attend the program, and therefore, it was concluded that the repeat programs increased physical performance and slowed down the progression of the disease [11]. Two-third of COPD patients administered repeat PR program achieved significant improvement in exercise capacity. It seems offering repeat PR programs to COPD patients when necessary is beneficial even after a long time between interventions [12]. In severe COPD patients who attended PR programs for three times with 6-month intervals, dyspnea, fatigue and quality of life scores improved, and bed-days decreased after 1 year. No favorable changes were observed in patients who administered PR for once [13]. There were clinically significant improvements in exercise tolerance and quality of life in patients who repeated the PR program within 1–3 years; however, the increase in walk distance was less compared to the increase achieved after the first program. Thus, early intervention and a longer program are recommended [14].

Another method to reinforce and prolong the benefits of a successful rehabilitation program may be the maintenance programs after the program. However, optimal strategies have not yet been described to meet this goal [6]. There are different approaches about the exercise type, level of supervision, physiotherapy strategies, duration and frequency of administration in the maintenance program. Therefore, the effectiveness of maintenance program is debated for the moment [15]. Following the 8-week PR program administered to moderate and severe COPD patients, patients were provided with a similar home-based program for 3 years (15 min of chest physiotherapy, 30 min of arm exercise, and 30 min of leg exercise) and they were called by physiotherapists every 15 days. In patients assessed on years 1, 2 and 3, it was seen that the significant change in BODE index and walk distance disappeared after year 2 [15]. Similarly, in patients with moderate and severe COPD who took supervised daily exercise for 3 months and weekly supervised breathing exercises for 6 months following 3-month PR, it was determined that the positive improvements in dyspnea, fatigue, walk distance and quality of life substantially diminished after year 2 [16]. It was observed that the exercise tolerance increased in patients with chronic pulmonary disease who were called every week for 12 months and who took supervised reinforcement sessions once a month, they had an improved medical condition and that the duration of their stay in the hospital decreased, however those positive effects disappeared at the end of year 2. Besides, no changes were found in respiratory functions, perception of dyspnea, self-efficacy, quality of life and use of healthcare resources and the improvement provided by the maintenance treatment after PR was reported as mild [5]. According to a study where mild COPD patients with exercise intolerance were visited by physiotherapists for 20 months following a 4-month PR program, dyspnea, exercise capacity and quality of life changed favorably and that those benefits were maintained for 2 years [17]. In several other studies, it was suggested that maintenance treatment was useless in maintaining the benefits [18, 19]. COPD patients prescribed exercise to do at home after PR program attended an exercise support group once a month and contacted via telephone calls once a month. At the end of the first year, no significant improvements were achieved in the exercise capacity and quality of life of the patients [18]. In COPD patients provided with 1-h patient-tailored exercise training and 1-h education every 3 months, no positive changes were recorded at the end of 1 year and thus, it was indicated that maintenance program had no effect on maintaining the benefits and that other methods were required to achieve that [19].

Some studies went beyond the traditional methods and investigated the effectiveness of several technological devices [7]. Moderate and severe COPD patients were given auditory stimuli after PR and asked to walk for 30–45 min 2–5 times per week, and there had been a decrease in perception of dyspnea and a significant increase in walk distance at the end of week 8. Based on this result, it was indicated that giving auditory stimuli was both a simple and a cost effective method to increase the efficiency of maintenance treatment after PR. Use of motion-sensitive devices during and after the program had been a research subject [20, 21]. No difference was detected between COPD patients using pedometer during and for 6 months after 8-week PR program and the patients who did not use the device in terms of physical activity [20]. When accelerometers were used in severe and very severe COPD patients attended to PR program, although there were no changes in unsupervised exercises, it was observed that physical activity in supervised exercises increased. Therefore, it is important to use an accelerometer to measure the walking habit and daily activity of COPD patients with severe dyspnea [21]. To see the changes in physical activity, a sensitive, valid and reliable accelerometer pedometer should be preferred [7].

In brief, it is not enough to increase the exercise capacity, decrease the perception of dyspnea and to improve the quality of live in patients after PR. In order to maintain these benefits, it is required to increase the physical activities of the patients and change the lifestyle of the patients at the end of the program. In most of the studies on this matter, it was found that the improvement in quality of life continued and the diseases progression slowed through repeat programs although the decrease in perception of dyspnea and increase in exercise capacity were not maintained. While it was shown that the benefits were maintained for 2 years with maintenance programs, the type of exercise, frequency of supervision and the length of program are not clear yet; therefore, there is are no recommended maintenance programs. A very small number of studies related to the use of technological devices suggested that giving auditory stimuli or using accelerometer during and after the program had an impact on increasing the physical activity.

Author details

Hulya Sahin
Dr. Surat Seren Chest Diseases and Thoracic Surgery Training and Research Hospital, Pulmonary Rehabilitation Unit, Izmir, Turkey

*Address all correspondence to: drhdogan@yahoo.com

References

[1] Hill K, Bansal V, Brooks D, Goldstein RS. Repeat pulmonary rehabilitation programs confer similar increases in functional exercise capacity to initial programs. Journal of Cardiopulmonary Rehabilitation and Prevention. 2008;**28**:410-414

[2] Nici L, Donner C, Wouters E, Zuwallack R, Ambrosino N, Bourbeau J, et al. American Thoracic Society/European Respiratory Society statement on pulmonary rehabilitation. American Journal of Respiratory and Critical Care Medicine. 2006;**173**:1390-1413

[3] Bauldoff GS, Hoffman LA, Zullo TG, Sciurba FC. Exercise maintenance following pulmonary rehabilitation: Effect of distractive stimuli. Chest. 2002;**122**:948-954

[4] Egan C, Deering BM, Blake C, Fullen BM, McCormack NM, Spruit MA, et al. Short term and long term effects of pulmonary rehabilitation on physical activity in COPD. Respiratory Medicine. 2012;**106**:1671-1679

[5] Ries AL, Kaplan RM, Myers R, Prewitt LM. Maintenance after pulmonary rehabilitation in chronic lung disease: A randomized trial. American Journal of Respiratory and Critical Care Medicine. 2003;**167**:880-888

[6] Corhay JL, Dang DN, Van Cauwenberge H, Louis R. Pulmonary rehabilitation and COPD: Providing patients a good environment for optimizing therapy. International Journal of Chronic Obstructive Pulmonary Disease. 2014;**9**:27-39

[7] Cindy Ng LW, Mackney J, Jenkins S, Hill K. Does exercise training change physical activity in people with COPD? A systematic review and meta-analysis. Chronic Respiratory Disease. 2012;**9**:17-26

[8] Pitta F, Troosters T, Probst VS, Langer D, Decramer M, Gosselink R. Are patients with COPD more active after pulmonary rehabilitation? Chest. 2008;**134**:273-280

[9] Jácome C, Marques A. Short- and long-term effects of pulmonary rehabilitation in patients with mild COPD: A comparison with patients with moderate to severe COPD. Journal of Cardiopulmonary Rehabilitation and Prevention. 2016;**36**:445-453

[10] Foglio K, Bianchi L, Ambrosino N. Is it really useful to repeat outpatient pulmonary rehabilitation programs in patients with chronic airway obstruction? A 2-year controlled study. Chest. 2001;**119**:1696-1704

[11] Stav D, Raz M, Shpirer I. Three years of pulmonary rehabilitation: Inhibit the decline in airflow obstruction, improves exercise endurance time, and body-mass index, in chronic obstructive pulmonary disease. BMC Pulmonary Medicine. 2009;**9**:26

[12] Atabaki A, Fine J, Haggerty M, Marolda C, Wakefield D, Yu A, et al. Effectiveness of repeated courses of pulmonary rehabilitation on functional exercise capacity in patients with COPD. Journal of Cardiopulmonary Rehabilitation and Prevention. 2015;**35**:272-277

[13] Romagnoli M, Dell'Orso D, Lorenzi C, Crisafulli E, Costi S, Lugli D, et al. Repeated pulmonary rehabilitation in severe and disabled COPD patients. Respiration. 2006;**73**:769-776

[14] Heng H, Lee AL, Holland AE. Repeating pulmonary rehabilitation: Prevalence, predictors and outcomes. Respirology. 2014;**19**:999-1005

[15] Güell MR, Cejudo P, Ortega F, Puy MC, Rodríguez-Trigo G, Pijoan JI,

et al. Benefits of long-term pulmonary rehabilitation maintenance program in patients with severe chronic obstructive pulmonary disease. Three-year follow-up. American Journal of Respiratory and Critical Care Medicine. 2017;**195**:622-629

[16] Güell R, Casan P, Belda J, Sangenis M, Morante F, Guyatt GH, et al. Long-term effects of outpatient rehabilitation of COPD: A randomized trial. Chest. 2000;**117**:976-983

[17] van Wetering CR, Hoogendoorn M, Mol SJ, Rutten-van Mölken MP, Schols AM. Short- and long-term efficacy of a community-based COPD management programme in less advanced COPD: A randomised controlled trial. Thorax. 2010;**65**:7-13

[18] Brooks D, Krip B, Mangovski-Alzamora S, Goldstein RS. The effect of postrehabilitation programmes among individuals with chronic obstructive pulmonary disease. The European Respiratory Journal. 2002;**20**:20-29

[19] Wilson AM, Browne P, Olive S, Clark A, Galey P, Dix E, et al. The effects of maintenance schedules following pulmonary rehabilitation in patients with chronic obstructive pulmonary disease: A randomised controlled trial. BMJ Open. 2015;**5**:e005921

[20] Nolan CM, Maddocks M, Canavan JL, Jones SE, Delogu V, Kaliaraju D, et al. Pedometer step count targets during pulmonary rehabilitation in chronic obstructive pulmonary disease. A randomized controlled trial. American Journal of Respiratory and Critical Care Medicine. 2017;**195**:1344-1352

[21] Steele BG, Belza B, Hunziker J, Holt L, Legro M, Coppersmith J, et al. Monitoring daily activity during pulmonary rehabilitation using a triaxial accelerometer. Journal of Cardiopulmonary Rehabilitation. 2003;**23**:139-142

Section 5

Thorax Surgery

Chapter 8

The Realm of Oncological Lung Surgery: From Past to Present and Future Perspectives

Alexander Maat, Amir Hossein Sadeghi, Ad Bogers and Edris Mahtab

Abstract

In this chapter, a historical overview as well as an overview of state of the art of the surgical techniques for the treatment of lung cancer is outlined. The chapter focuses on the introduction of open surgery, video-assisted thoracic surgery (VATS), uniportal VATS (UVATS), and robotic-assisted thoracic surgery (RATS) techniques for lung resections. A short introduction on upcoming techniques and modalities is given. The currently available tools as three-dimensional (3D) computed tomography (CT), virtual reality, and endo-bronchial surgery will be discussed. Based on the current development, this chapter attempts to delineate the horizon of oncological lung surgery. The information is generated not only from the available literature, but also from the experiences of surgeons and other physicians as well as co-workers involved in lung cancer treatment around the world. This chapter can be seen as a general introduction to several aspects of oncological lung surgery.

Keywords: lung cancer, lung surgery, VATS, UVATS, RATS, thoracotomy, virtual reality, endo-bronchial surgery

1. Introduction

For centuries, the inside of the chest cavity was a no-go area for complex surgical interventions. The problems of an open pneumothorax were already known by the ancient Greek Celsus around the year 30 AD noted: “as soon as the knife really penetrates to the chest, by cutting through the transverse septum, a sort of membrane which divides the upper from the lower parts, the man loses his life at once” [1].

At that time, drainage of an empyema as described by Hippocrates (approx. 460–375 BC) was the only feasible operation [2]. The first report of a successful lung resection is attributed to Roland of Parma in 1499 who resected the herniating part of a lung, days after a penetrating chest trauma [3]. In 1846, general anesthesia with ether had been introduced by William Morton in Boston, an extremely important step in the history of surgery.

During the mid-nineteenth century, when tuberculosis reached its highest incidence, it was recognized that a state of rigidity of the mediastinum permitted an open pneumothorax. Estlander of Helsingfors was one of the first to describe wide thoracoplasty in order to “rest” a lung affected by tuberculosis (“decostalisation of the chest” in 1879) [4].

IntechOpen

During the late nineteenth century, many experiments were carried out, mainly in animals, aimed at performing lobectomy and pneumonectomy. Usually these experiments were done in stages, the first procedure aiming at creating a state of fixation of the mediastinum. The world still was not ready yet for primary lung resections.

Further in this chapter, a historical overview and an overview of modern surgical techniques for the treatment of lung cancer are outlined. The focus is on the introduction of open surgery as well as the minimally invasive surgery. In addition, a short introduction to upcoming techniques and modalities is given.

2. The evolution of thoracic surgery: a journey through time

2.1 The first giant steps: aseptic approach, X-ray, and positive pressure ventilation

During the late nineteenth century, Joseph Lister, based on Louis Pasteur's theory of micro-organisms, introduced the concept of asepsis in 1867. Surgeon's hands, instruments, and surgical wounds were sterilized with 5% carbolic acid (phenol) solution and a mist of phenol was sprayed into the surgical field [5]. This policy led to an extreme reduction of post-operative mortality and for this reason, Lister is regarded as the father of modern surgery. Caroline Hampton, chief nurse and later on the wife of William Halsted, one of the founding fathers of the John's Hopkins Hospital, developed severe dermatitis due to frequent exposure to phenol and mercuric chloride. This provoked Halsted to ask the Goodyear Company to develop rubber gloves to protect the hands of the surgical team. These became available at the end of 1890 and were soon used throughout the world [6].

The aftermath of the nineteenth century saw the discovery of X-ray by William Konrad Rontgen in 1895. For the first time in mankind, it became possible to identify large tumors in the chest when not shaded by the heart and other mediastinal structures. At the turn of the twentieth century, the major barrier to enable one stage intrathoracic surgery was that of the open pneumothorax. This is remarkable since the anatomist Vesalius in 1543 had extensively studied respiration and already studied tracheotomy and positive pressure ventilation. His ideas would be dormant for about 3.5 centuries [7]. Based on this concept that there should be a pressure difference between the intra-alveolar pressure and the atmospheric pressure, Sauerbruch, still an assistant of von Mikulicz, developed the negative pressure chamber [8]—a genius idea, but quite unpractical. Only two of these operation theaters were built worldwide, one in Germany and the other one in the German Hospital (today the Lenox-Hill hospital) in New York where the surgeon Willy Meyer, emigrated to the USA from Germany in 1884, added a small positive pressure chamber over the patients head in 1909, this was called the super chamber but it was never clinically used [9]. Willy Meyer would become one of the founding fathers of the American Association for Thoracic Surgery (AATS) in 1918.

In the same year, 1909, and also in New York, Meltzer and his son-in-law Auer launched their concept of positive pressure ventilation, using a flexible silk woven tracheal catheter and a continuous stream of air mixed with ether [10]. Their concept was the birth of modern anesthesia. Recognizing that this was an enormous step forward, Meltzer was invited to become the first president of the AATS. In a speech delivered at the founding meeting of the AATS, Willy Meyers stated: "The thorax was the last fortress to be attacked and it has been laid open safely to the surgeon's knife" [9].

2.2 Smoking induced global lung cancer epidemic

Lung cancer was a very rare disease in the beginning of the twentieth century. In 1919, Alton Ochsner, as a medical student was invited with his whole class to witness an autopsy of a patient who died of lung cancer. The pathologist announced that no one in that class would ever again see another such case [11]. It took 17 years before Ochsner, who had become a surgeon, saw his second case, followed by 8 other cases in the 6 following months. All of these patients were male and had served as soldiers in World War I and in the line of duty they had taken up the habit of smoking, provoked by mass advertisements promoting smoking. Ochsner was amongst the first surgeons to correlate smoking to the development of lung cancer [12]. With the lung cancer epidemic which started after World War I, the number of patients with potentially resectable lung cancer increased significantly. Two major surgical items had to be settled; should a lung resection for cancer be a lobectomy or a pneumonectomy and what is the best surgical technique? Is it mass hilar ligation or anatomical dissection? The first report on lobectomy for lung cancer was that of Edward Churchill (Boston) in 1932 [13]. One year later, Evarts Graham, while intending to perform a lobectomy, was forced to perform a pneumonectomy because the tumor was very centrally located in the hilum at the origin of the left upper lobe (bronchoplastic procedures such as sleeve resection had not been developed yet) [14]. For a considerably long period, pneumonectomy was regarded as the golden standard for all lung cancer patients. Lobectomy by many was considered inferior and compared with lumpectomy without resection of loco-regional lymph nodes in breast cancer [15]. Only in 1962, a large case series between pneumonectomy and lobectomy were compared showing that lobectomy was equivalent to pneumonectomy as a cancer operation but with a lower rate of complications and mortality [16].

2.3 Fundamental steps in the development of state-of-the-art lung surgery

With respect to surgical technique, there was no consensus on hilar control; mass ligation or anatomical dissection and step-by-step control of the hilar structures. Cadaveric studies performed by Blades and Kent in the early 1940s pushed the world toward the latter, later supported by several publications of Boyes on the intrahilar anatomy of the lung segments [10, 17].

With this knowledge, Clement Thomas Price (London, 1947) introduced the concept of parenchyma sparing operations, having done the first anatomical segmentectomy in a lung cancer patient [18]. The first sleeve resection for bronchogenic carcinoma was performed in 1952 [19]. Consequently, it was around the mid-1950s the four main operations in lung cancer as we know today were in the armamentarium of the thoracic surgeon: pneumonectomy, lobectomy, sleeve lobectomy, and segmentectomy.

A major step forward was the introduction of double lumen endo-tracheal tube by Carlens in 1949 [20]. With this selective single lung ventilation concept, modern lung surgery is greatly facilitated, particularly, the endoscopic and robotic techniques used nowadays (discussed later in this chapter).

Diagnostic techniques were still very primitive in that era compared with today's standards. Besides standard chest X-ray, there was rigid bronchoscopy, bronchography, planography, and cytology. The concept of staging had to be developed yet. Exploratory thoracotomy in "operable patients" was performed with a very low threshold, not to lose time. Some authors reported up to 50% inoperability [21]. In the Amsterdam University Hospital between 1955 and 1960 in a series of 100 exploratory thoracotomies in patients who were found to be inoperable, 54% of patients had complications and 9 of the 100 patients died due to post-operative complications [22]. In 63% of the cases, mediastinal ingrowth or large irresectable nodes were found. In 23%, there was in growth in heart and/or major vessels, 12% ingrowth into the thoracic wall, 1% in growth in the diaphragm, and 1% pleural carcinomatosis. By far, mediastinal involvement was the leading cause of inoperability. In 1959, Carlens had published his experience with 100 mediastinoscopies [20]. The morbidity of this technique was 2.5% and the mortality was less than 0.5%, way better then exploratory thoracotomy. The Amsterdam team embraced mediastinoscopy and combined this in a series of operable patients with bronchoscopy and on indication diagnostic pneumothorax. Due to the mediastinoscopy findings, the resection rate in Amsterdam rose from 60 to 94% with 12% false positive mediastinoscopies [20]. Years later, in 1984, Griffith Pearson published a landmark paper showing that when positive mediastinal nodes were found, any subsequent lung resection would not cure a patient [23].

The world was waiting for methods to better identify loco-regional progression and distant metastases. Hounsfield, by combining tomography images with the calculating power of a computer, constructed the first computed tomography (CT) scanner, first for brain scans only, but in 1975 he and his team built the first whole body scanner. The computed tomography (CT) scanner was soon to be followed by the magnetic resonance imaging (MRI) scanner in 1977, while the next big step was the combination of positron emission tomography (PET) and CT scanners in 1991. The use of mediastinoscopy has declined after the introduction of ultrasound-guided examinations of the mediastinum and the hilum (endo-esophageal ultrasound (EUS) and endo-bronchial ultrasound bronchoscopy (EBUS)), but is still used on a regular base when the latter techniques fall short.

2.4 The rise of minimally invasive lung surgery

For decades, postero-lateral thoracotomy has been the preferred entrance for most lung resections (**Figure 1A**). However, the price of an excellent exposure to the lung hilum came with high percentages of long standing post-operative pain, discomfort, and functional loss.

The Swedish internist Jacobeus is often positioned as the founding father of thoracoscopy but in fact, it was the British surgeon Francis Richard Cruse who already had published this technique in 1865 [24].

The first thoracoscopic resections were not immediately embraced by the surgical community. Ralph Lewis was the first one to publish a series of 100 lobectomies done thoracoscopically [25]. Lacking experience, tailor-made instruments, and specific endo-staplers, these resections were performed using a mass stapling technique. In Los Angeles, Robert McKenna worked out a standardized approach for video-assisted thoracic surgery (VATS) lobectomy (**Figure 1B**), working through the hilum from anterior to posterior; in 2006, he published a series of 1100 cases [26].

This provoked surgeons around the world to adapt this technique and today in many hospitals, it is the preferred approach for the majority of cases. In 2019, Eric Lim published the results of the VIOLET trial, a prospective randomized trial between VATS and thoracotomy in lung cancer patients. VATS showing to be superior with respect to major adverse events, less pain on post-operative day 2 and shorter median hospital stay with an equal oncological outcome (number of lymph nodes harvested and upstaged and R-0 resections) [27].

Studies on chronic pain (pain for which patients visit a doctor 3 months post-operative), however, did not show a major difference in pain between thoracotomy

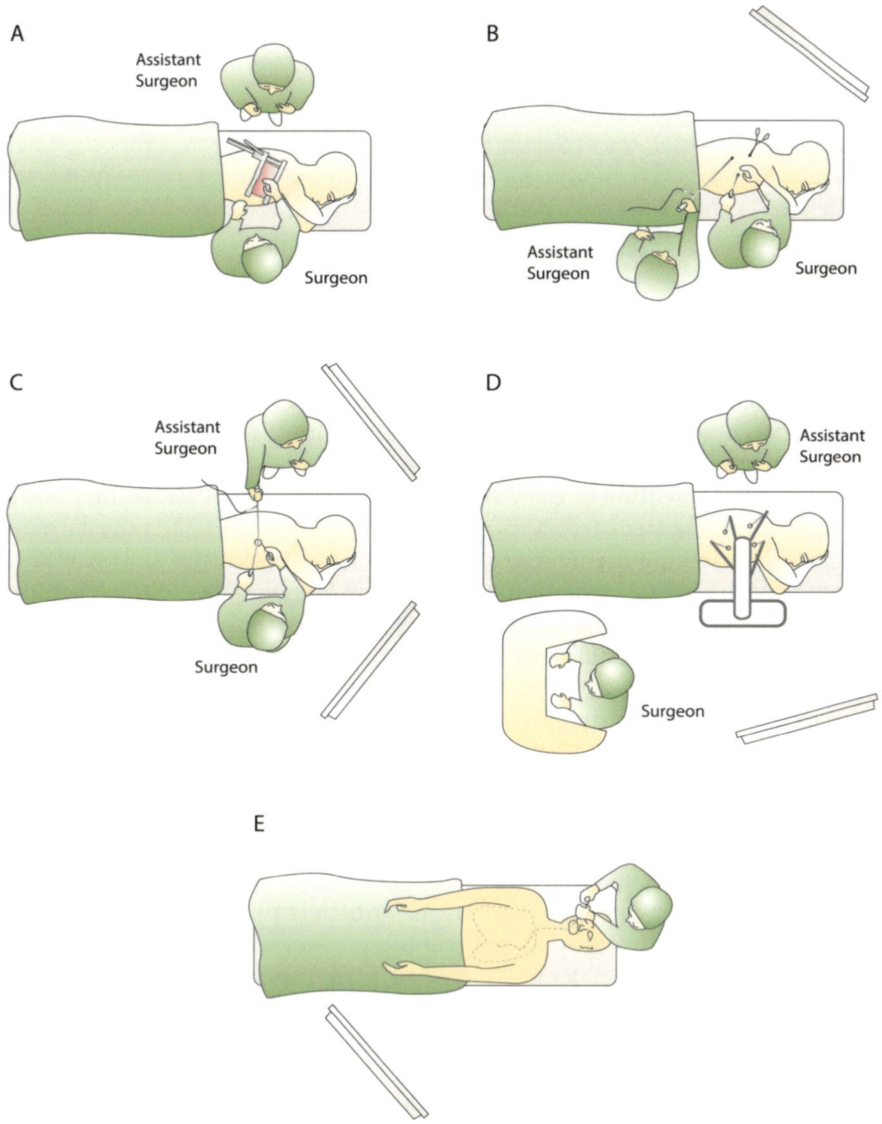

Figure 1.
Overview of the surgical approaches for treatment of lung cancer. (A) Postero-lateral thoracotomy, (B) 3 ports, video-assisted thoracic surgery (VATS), (C) uniportal video-assisted thoracic surgery (UVATS), (D) robotic-assisted thoracic surgery (RATS), and (E) endo-bronchial surgery.

patients and VATS patients 3–6 months post-operatively [28]. Chronic pain after VATS is often contributed to the insult of multiple intercostal nerves by trocars and instruments. It has to be seen whether the explanation is that simple, however, it moved surgeons to search for even less invasive methods, eventually leading to the concept of uniportal VATS (UVATS), first proposed by Rocco in 2004 [29] (**Figure 1C**).

There is still no proof that an UVATS approach leads to less pain, discomfort, and loss of functionality compared with multiple port VATS.

With the idea of intercostal nerve damage in mind, surgeons have also explored other VATS-assisted intrathoracic pathways like subxiphoid and cervical approaches [30, 31]. Others are exploring a hybrid approach, combining 5 mm intercostal ports with a subxiphoid approach [32].

Almost parallel with the introduction and evolution of VATS, the world saw the introduction of robotic-assisted thoracic surgery (RATS), first published by Franca Melfi and her team [33] (**Figure 1D**).

Up till now, no significant differences have been shown in complications and outcome between VATS, UVATS, and RATS [34]. The major reason that the introduction of RATS lagged behind in many institutions is a financial reason; it is not cost-efficient. In the meantime, VATS has evolutionized to three-dimensional VATS (3D VATS) and robotic-like instruments have become available for laparoscopic and VATS procedures.

2.4.1 Sub-lobar resection: the rise of segmentectomy

During the last decade, there is a growing interest in lung parenchyma-sparing resections. This need is more highlighted by the results of the two largest population based national screening studies (NLST, 2011 and NELSON, 2018) showing that discovery and resection of early stage lung cancer through screening programs lead to significantly better survival of patients [35, 36]. The NLST study showed a reduction of 20% in lung cancer mortality for annual screening over 3 years with low-dose CT with a greater benefit for screening in women. The NELSON study showed for screening with low-dose CT, a 26% reduction of lung cancer mortality in high-risk men and up to 61% reduction of lung cancer mortality in high-risk women over a 10-year period. Nowadays, there is a trend toward sub-lobar resection as segmentectomy, making the oncological lung surgery even more challenging. Moreover, this makes the role of peri-operative diagnostic tools as fluorescent indocyanine green (ICG) [37], 3D-CT modalities, and (navigational) bronchoscopy interventions (next section, **Figure 1E**) indispensable. Because of its anatomical complexity, many surgeons hesitate to perform segmentectomy. For this reason, in 2012, Hiroaki Nomori and Morihito Okada published the book "Illustrated Anatomical Segmentectomy for Lung Cancer" which is an essential book for surgeons starting a segmentectomy program at their centers. In 2019, segmentectomy is mostly performed in countries of Eastern Asia, such as Japan, followed by few centers in the USA and Western Europe.

3. Advances in thoracic imaging facilitating minimally invasive lung surgery: a brief outlook into the future

Over the past few decades, imaging modalities such as CT, PET-CT, and standard chest X-ray imaging have played a key role in the non-invasive diagnostic work-up of thoracic disease. In addition, these imaging modalities are an essential part of the preoperative planning process of thoracic surgical procedures. Even though there is a broad range of clinical indications for various thoracic imaging modalities and the information provided by all different modalities is different, the purpose of this section is not to undertake a comprehensive evaluation of the characteristics of these imaging modalities. Specifically, this section will focus on innovative preoperative and intraoperative imaging modalities as a surgical planning and navigation tools and provide a brief overview of new developments in medical imaging, especially in the context of (oncologic) pulmonary resections.

3.1 Three-dimensional computed tomography (3D-CT)

In the setting of oncologic thoracic surgery, a standard chest CT scan can be used to evaluate the extensiveness of disease in terms of pleural, mediastinal, chest wall, or vascular involvement. In addition, the CT scan is used to study the surgical anatomy of the pulmonary artery (and its major branches), pulmonary vein, and bronchial structures when a resection of the lung parenchyma is planned. Due to the establishment and development of more modern multislice CT scanners, it has become easier to detect smaller peripheral tumors. While this has enabled more diagnostic accuracy, it has resulted in an increased clinical use of sublobar anatomic resections. Specifically, in the setting of anatomic segmental pulmonary resections, which are technically and anatomically more demanding and complex, there is a need for more accurate imaging modalities that enables better preoperative knowledge of the surgical anatomy (such as bronchial and vascular anatomy in sublobar/segmental levels). Recently, an increasing number of scientific reports have been published on the use of preoperative three-dimensional (3D)-CT reconstruction as a surgical planning tool before anatomic resection of pulmonary segments or lobes [38–42]. According to some of these studies, the preoperative use of 3D-CT reconstructed images is feasible and safe and, in some cases, associated with shorter operative time due to better preoperative understanding of surgical anatomy [38, 42]. In order to obtain 3D-CT image reconstructions, different methods are described and various (free open-source) software packets are available [42–44]. However, there are also limitations regarding the utility of software to reconstruct 3D images of CT scans. For example, the identification and separation of the pulmonary artery and vein may be a challenging and time-consuming process. Moreover, in some cases, a contrast-enhanced CT scan is required to create 3D-simulations, which increases the risks of radiation exposure. In addition, the reconstruction commonly requires technical support and the assistance of radiology and information and communication technology (ICT) experts.

Oizumi et al. reported a study on the use of 3D reconstruction of multidetector CT (MDCT) images in order to plan and guide pulmonary segmentectomy preoperatively and during surgery [38]. It was noted that after the introduction of 3D-CT reconstruction, the number of (fairly) difficult classified segmentectomies that have been performed increased significantly, suggesting that preoperative 3D-CT simulation contributes fairly to the efficacy of surgical planning of complex segmentectomies. In addition, in a retrospective analysis of patients undergoing thoracoscopic segmentectomy reported by Xue et al., the authors found that when preoperative 3D-CT reconstruction was used to make operation plans, in 19% of the cases, the operation plan was changed due to the results of 3D simulation [42]. The original surgical plan of these cases was changed due to the expectation of an inadequate resection margin distance, based on pre-operative simulation results. This indicates that preoperative 3D simulation not only contributes to technical feasibility and efficacy of surgery, but also to the decision-making process from an oncological point of view.

Even though an increasing number of studies on the use of 3D-CT simulation are being published, the majority of them do not report on the differences in parameters of clinical outcome (such as perioperative blood loss, post-operative stay, and conversion rates to thoracotomy) but focus more on technical aspects and feasibility of 3D-simulation and surgery. However, the majority of reports do recognize the following advantages of preoperative 3D-simulation in the context of (sub-)lobar pulmonary resection: (1) classification and identification of anatomical (vascular and bronchial) abnormalities; (2) identification of unsuitable surgical cases for segmentectomy; (3) training of less experienced thoracic surgeons and surgical residents; (4) preoperative estimation of proper surgical resection margin; (5) a stepwise preoperative surgical planning; and (6) intraoperative navigation for identification of anatomical structures [38, 40–42].

3D-CT-mediated preoperative surgical planning and intraoperative guidance of (oncological) pulmonary surgery could contribute significantly to the development of more accurate and safer (sublobar) anatomic resections. In the near future, this technology will become more common in thoracic surgery. However, in order to reach that stage, some (mostly technical) limitations need to be overcome.

3.2 Virtual reality, augmented reality, and mixed reality

Virtual reality (VR) is a technology that enables users to interact with a computer-generated virtual 3D interface (**Figure 2**). More interestingly, in augmented reality (AR), the user is able to overlay aspects of the VR world within the real physical world. Finally, mixed reality (MR) allows users to create a hybrid physical and virtual world and offers the possibility to interact and analyze objects in the physical world by virtual projections [45, 46].

Recently, surgical intraoperative navigation as well as preoperative surgical simulation based on VR, MR, and AR have been developed and successfully used in various surgical fields including neurosurgery, liver surgery, kidney surgery, and orthopedic surgery [47–51]. In contrast to 2D interfaces (e.g. conventional CT scans), VR, MR, and AR enable not only visualization of anatomical structures but also allow interactive manipulation of the digital information (e.g. anatomic structures) provided by (wearable) computer-integrated devices (such as the Microsoft Hololens or the Google Glass). It has been suggested that these new interfaces might have the potential to benefit both the surgeon and the patient. For surgeons, this benefit comes by the way of improved preoperative surgical planning, better and more accurate intraoperative imaging guidance, and a better preoperative awareness of anatomical abnormalities. Patients will potentially benefit from shorter operative time, shorter length of hospital stay, and improved outcomes. Additionally, AR, VR, and MR offer the possibility to simulate surgical situations as well as facilitating training for surgeons and residents. In the field of thoracic surgery, some of these modalities have been used over the past few years in order to train surgical residents and surgeons to master the techniques necessary for minimally invasive lung surgery [52].

However, only very few reports are available on the use of AR, VR, or MR for surgical planning or intraoperative navigation for lung surgery [53–55]. Frajhof

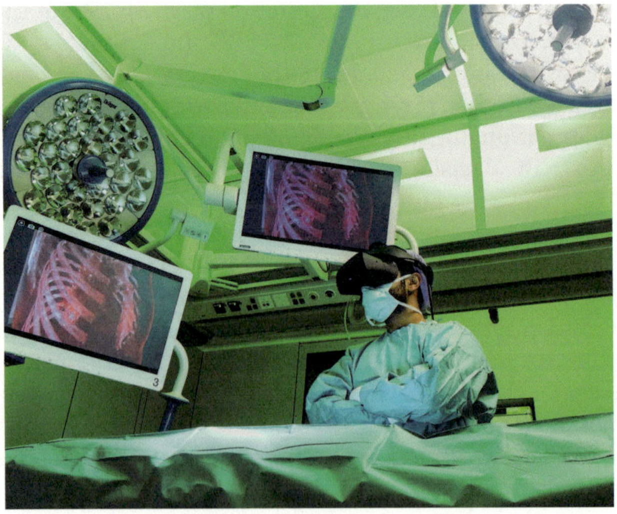

Figure 2.
An example of virtual reality application during minimally invasive lung cancer surgery in the operating theater.

et al. recently published a study on the use of AR, VR, and MR technology in the preoperative planning of a technically demanding VATS left upper lobectomy [53]. In another study from Rouzé et al., augmented reality was used as a navigation tool in combination with cone beam CT (CBCT) to guide intraoperative localization of pulmonary nodules for wedge resection through VATS. The investigators firstly localized the lesions by CBCT intraoperatively. Subsequently, a 3D reconstruction of the nodule was created by using software. After this, an augmented fluoroscopic 3D image of the pulmonary nodule was projected on a screen in front of the operating table. By this, the surgeon was able to localize the lesion intraoperatively and perform a wedge resection safely [54].

Interestingly, also some reports are available on the use of VR 3D reconstruction of the airways, known as virtual bronchoscopy, specifically used as a diagnostic aid tool in the assessment of airway masses and stenosis [56, 57]. Virtual bronchoscopy contributes fairly to the diagnostic process since it enables diagnostic maneuvers, such as assessing bronchial anatomy distally from stenoses, which are not possible with standard flexible bronchoscopy. Moreover, virtual bronchoscopy is a noninvasive method and does not bear any additional risks (e.g. radiation exposure or iatrogenic airway damage) for patients. Despite these advantages, virtual bronchoscopy is not expected to completely replace flexible bronchoscopy due to some limitations. For example, tumor boundaries can be misjudged by intrabronchial secretions that might lead to a false-positive result. Moreover, it has shown not to be sensitive and effective enough for detecting small mucosal abnormalities (e.g. erythema and erosion), dynamic stenoses (caused by, for example, the respiratory cycle or vocal cords), and in differentiating mucus plugs from a mass. Finally, virtual bronchoscopy has the limitation that it does not enable biopsies.

4. Advances in the armamentarium of (the endo-bronchial) lung cancer surgery

In the past two decades, there has been an increase in the development of innovative technologies to facilitate more accurate, efficient, and safe (minimally invasive) thoracic interventions. Specifically, there have been some reports on the progress of innovative therapeutic modalities that approach lung cancer through other minimally invasive methods than direct surgery. Examples of these therapeutic options are thermal ablation, including radiofrequency ablation (RFA), microwave ablation (MWA), and cryoablation of malignant lung lesions. This section will touch on some of these developments and review some outcomes of thermal ablation therapy.

4.1 Thermal ablation therapy

4.1.1 Radiofrequency ablation (RFA)

Amongst various thermal ablation therapies, RFA is a well-studied method, especially in the treatment of liver cancer [58, 59]. Due to favorable outcomes in the treatment of liver cancer, specifically hepatocellular carcinoma, the application of this technology to malignant lesions in other organs, including the lungs, has been growing. RFA involves the insertion of a probe inside the affected target tissue. The electrode on the probe generates frictional heat that creates coagulation necrosis of the surrounding (tumor) lung parenchyma. In pulmonary surgery, the use of RFA has been reported in the treatment of various malignant lesions including inoperable lung cancer [60–62], primary or metastatic pulmonary tumors of less than 3.5 cm in size [63], and stage I-4 non-small cellular lung cancer (NSCLC) not eligible for surgery [64–67]. Results from retrospective studies on RFA of primary malignant lung lesions have suggested reasonable overall 1-year survival rates ranging from 78 to 94% in patients with early stage lung cancer [66, 68–70]. A 5-year survival rates have been reported to be significantly lower and in the range of 25–58% [66, 71, 72]. Important prognostic factors in RFA therapy of lung cancer, in terms of survival, are the additional use of targeted systemic therapies, lesions less than 3 cm (diameter), a Charlson comorbidity index (an index of associated comorbidities) >5, and lower stage disease [66, 73].

A major drawback of RFA therapy compared with surgical resection is the poor results of local progression control [74]. This limitation might be explained by the fact that in RFA therapy no systematic lymph node dissection is carried out and, additionally, no good method exists to check for local adequate treatment margins. With regard to complications, pneumothorax is one of the most common complications associated with RFA. However, it is most often (>80%) treated conservatively without the need for chest tube drainage [75]. In addition, pleural effusion might develop after RFA, however, similar to pneumothorax, does not often (<5%) require intervention [75]. In summary, RFA therapy seems an effective and relatively safe intervention for treating lung cancer, however, a careful patient selection is necessary. Moreover, more future long-term and large randomized controlled trials are necessary to compare the clinical outcomes between RFA, surgical resection, and other modalities of thermal ablation therapy.

4.1.2 Microwave ablation (MWA)

MWA involves hyperthermia-mediated ablation of tissue by causing friction between water molecules in the target tissue. By creating a dipole excitation, hyperthermia is generated and coagulation necrosis results in the lesion and surrounding tissue [76, 77]. The placement of the probes is commonly guided by CT/CT-fluoroscopy. MWA has been successfully used to create larger ablation zones than RFA. Compared with RFA, MWA technology is thought to be more effective in creating larger zones of coagulation necrosis due to the elimination of heat loss through heat sink (the loss of heat through blood flow inside the target tissue) [76].

Studies and long-term data after MWA as a thermal ablation modality are limited when compared with RFA. In a recent review, Yuan and colleagues reported a meta-analysis of clinical outcomes after RFA and MWA for primary and metastatic pulmonary malignancies [75]. The authors identified 11 studies based on MWA compared with 42 studies based on RFA therapy, all with a retrospective study design. In this meta-analysis, it was demonstrated that RFA seems to be superior to MWA with regard to overall survival (up to 5 years) for both primary and metastatic pulmonary malignancies. However, the authors note that the results of lung metastasis should be interpreted carefully, since small groups of patients were included in the analysis based on only a few retrospective studies. With regard to local tumor progression free survival, RFA and MWA showed similar results. In addition, similar to RFA, MWA is a relatively safe intervention which is not associated with high complication rates. Yuan et al. reported comparable rates of pneumothorax and pleural effusion after ablation by MWA and RFA [75]. Concerning prognostic factors negatively affecting survival and local tumor progression control, more advanced disease stage, tumors >3 cm (diameter), and emphysematous lungs have been identified [78].

4.1.3 Cryoablation

An opposite method of hyperthermia induced ablation, termed cryoablation, creates protein denaturation, ischemia, cell rupture, and necrosis through local hypothermia (temperatures < −40°C) [79]. In this technique, compressed argon gas is used to create freezing temperatures that induce local injury to the tissue. Subsequently, helium is used to thaw the tissue. Comparable to MWA, in cryoablation, multiple probes can be used to increase the ablation area in the tissue and placement under the guidance of CT/CT-fluoroscopy. Although cryosurgery is a relatively old ablative technique, use of cryoablation in the context of lung cancer and long-term studies are limited. Besides percutaneous cryoablation, other methods of cryoablative strategies are endo-bronchial (for obstructive intrabronchial tumors) (**Figure 1E**) and intrathoracic (during surgery). Specific indications for each modality have been reviewed by Niu and colleagues and are beyond the scope of this chapter [80].

Since thermal ablation therapies are commonly reserved for patients not eligible for curative surgery, tumor recurrence after radiotherapy or patients who refuse surgery, even though they have resectable lesions, cryoablation is often offered as a therapy to palliate symptoms or to increase survival in advanced disease stage. Consequently, a number of reports have been published on the use of cryoablation for the treatment of medically inoperable NSCLC, advanced stages of NSCLC, and for pulmonary metastasis [80–84]. Niu et al. reported on a series of 840 patients with NSCLC who received percutaneous cryoablative therapy for various stages of NSCLC ranging from IIa to IV. The reported overall survival was 68, 52, 34, 26, and 17% for 1-, 2-, 3-, 4-, and 5-year, respectively. Local and peripheral recurrence rates were 28.3 and 47.2%, respectively, after a median follow-up of 34 months (range 4–63 months). For patients with less advanced NSCLC, better outcome is reported in terms of overall survival. In 2012, Yamauchi et al. demonstrated a 2-year overall survival of 88% in medically inoperable patients with stage I NSCLC who were treated with percutaneous cryoablation [84]. In addition, Moore and colleagues published a study in which an overall survival rate of 67.8% was reported in patients with stage I NSCLC after 5 years [82].

Regarding cryoablation therapy in metastatic lung lesions, studies have also proven the efficacy and safety of percutaneous cryoablation. For example, Yamauchi et al. reported a 3-year progression free survival rate of 59% for patients with metastatic colorectal carcinoma treated with cryoablation [85]. Factors associated with local tumor progression or poor prognosis have been studied by multivariate analyses. Interestingly, most of these factors (e.g. tumor size <3 cm and stage of disease) are comparable to the factors in other modalities of thermal ablation [78, 80]. Regarding the safety profile of cryoablation compared with other modalities of thermal ablation, comparable rates of pneumothorax and pleural effusion are reported in the literature [77, 80]. However, incidental reports of transient recurrent laryngeal nerve neuropraxia have also been documented [86].

5. Conclusions

Until the late nineteenth century, the inside of the chest cavity was a no-go area for complex surgical interventions. The world still was not ready yet for primary lung resections. To make the lung surgery possible, several giant steps were undertaken: the introduction of aseptic concept by Joseph Lister in 1867, the discovery of X-ray by William Konrad Rontgen in 1895, and the introduction of positive pressure ventilation by Meltzer and Auer in 1909. With the lung cancer epidemic after World War I, the number of patients with potentially resectable lung cancer increased significantly. Surgeons around the world were debating on the preferable resection (lobectomy vs. pneumonectomy) and the best surgical technique: mass hilar ligation versus anatomical dissection. While the first report on lobectomy for lung cancer in 1932, it took almost 30 years to report that lobectomy was the preferred resection for lung cancer surgery. In the same period, the anatomical dissection technique gained wider application. This all together with the discovery of double lumen endo-tracheal tube by Carlens in 1949 paved the way for modern lung resection techniques. The introduction of diagnostic tools as CT, MRI, PET-CT, and later EUS and EBUS facilitated even better tumor localization and mediastinal evaluation decreasing the surgical mortality.

The next major challenge was decreasing the morbidity of thoracotomy: high percentages of long standing post-operative pain, discomfort, and functional loss. The solution led to the development of modern minimally invasive lung surgery. In 2006, Robert McKenna published a standardized approach for VATS lobectomy in a series of 1100 cases leading to global adaptation of VATS for lung surgery. While VATS showing to be superior with respect to major adverse events, less pain on post-operative day 2 and shorter median hospital stay with an equal oncological outcome, studies on chronic pain, however, did not show a major difference in pain between thoracotomy and VATS. This moved surgeons to search for even less invasive methods, eventually leading to the concept of uniportal VATS, first proposed by Rocco in 2004, subxiphoid and cervical approaches, and hybrid approach combining 5 mm intercostal ports with a subxiphoid approach. At the same time, the world witnessed the introduction of RATS by Franca Melfi and her team, however, because of the financial reasons, the introduction of RATS in many centers lagged behind. In the meantime, VATS has evolutionized to 3D-VATS and robotic like instruments have become available for laparoscopic and VATS procedures. Whether all these approaches will lead to reduction of chronic pain is yet to be determined.

The results of major screening programs have shifted the trend of lung resection toward sub-lobar resection as segmentectomy, making the lung surgery even more challenging. Moreover, this makes the role of peri-operative imaging tools as fluorescent indocyanine green (ICG), 3D-CT modalities, and (navigational) bronchoscopy interventions indispensable.

The upcoming VR, AR, and MR enable a more naturalistic 3D presentation of human anatomy in a digital interface. As a diagnostic tool, it can provide physicians with a more realistic view of the patient's anatomy and might enable diagnostic assessment, preoperative surgical planning, and intraoperative guidance. In addition, it can provide training and learning platform for students, residents, and surgeons. It has already proven its added value for a broad range of surgical procedures; however, AR/VR/MR has not been used widely in thoracic surgery yet. Considering the speed of development of this technology in other areas, it is expected that it will make its way into the world of thoracic surgery in the near future. In this perspective, hybrid operating theaters including 3D-CT and (robotic-assisted) navigational bronchoscopy tools are already on their way. To address this, however, it is essential that thoracic surgeons have an active and open attitude toward the introduction of innovative (digital) applications.

With respect to endo-bronchial interventions, thermal ablation therapy seems to provide an efficacious and safe alternative for surgical therapy of lung cancer and lung cancer metastasis. However, patient's selection should be carried out with caution and should be personalized for each patient based on type of cancer (e.g. NSCLC), comorbidities, tumor size, and disease stage. Specifically, thermal ablation therapy could offer a palliative or even a life-prolonging treatment option for non-surgical candidates. Hopefully future long-term and larger prospective (randomized controlled) trials will answer the remaining questions. For example, it will be necessary to study the impact of combining thermal ablation therapy with other conventional (e.g. systemic or radiotherapy) therapies for the treatment of lung cancer. In addition, more data are warranted on the determination of the best therapy for incomplete ablations and/or local recurrence of disease. More interestingly, biomarkers or novel imaging techniques to follow-up on ablative therapies are also required, especially since the radiological follow-up of recently ablated lung tissue is very challenging. More data and confirmation of these data are therefore necessary and need to be generated by future multicenter trials.

To conclude, this chapter provides a historical overview and a summary of state-of-the-art surgical techniques in the treatment of lung cancer today. The journey of lung surgery was and is a very challenging one, with major hurdles to overcome. It departed from a "no-go" era, leaving behind the golden standard of pneumonectomy and thoracotomy, to arrive in the current era of minimally invasive and robotic-assisted surgery. The journey continues toward the horizon of non-intubated operations, sub-lobar resections, virtual reality imaging modalities, navigational bronchoscopy interventions, and hybrid procedures. We are heading toward the era of incisionless, natural orifice surgery: an almost science fiction vision, yet nothing is more real.

Acknowledgements

The contribution of Egied Simons (Simons Productions, Mathenesserdijk 236A, 3026 GL, Rotterdam, The Netherlands) and Chris Hordijk (Medical VR, van Eeghenstraat 98, 1071JL, Amsterdam, The Netherlands) in generating the figures is highly appreciated. We would like to thank Dr. F. Incekara (Departments of Neurosurgery and Radiology, Erasmus Medical Center, Rotterdam, The Netherlands) for his helpful advice.

Abbreviations

VATS	video-assisted thoracic surgery
UVATS	uniportal video-assisted thoracic surgery
RATS	robotic-assisted thoracic surgery
3D	three-dimensional
CT	computed tomography scanner
AATS	American Association for Thoracic Surgery
MRI	magnetic resonance imaging scanner
PET	positron emission tomography
EUS	endo-esophageal ultrasound
EBUS	endo-bronchial ultrasound bronchoscopy
ICG	indocyanine green
ICT	information and communication technology
MDCT	multidetector computed tomography
VR	virtual reality
AR	augmented reality
MR	mixed reality
CBCT	cone beam computed tomography
RFA	radiofrequency ablation
MWA	microwave ablation
NSCLC	non-small cellular lung cancer

Author details

Alexander Maat, Amir Hossein Sadeghi, Ad Bogers and Edris Mahtab*
Department of Cardio-thoracic Surgery, Erasmus Medical Centre, Erasmus University, Rotterdam, The Netherlands

*Address all correspondence to: e.mahtab@erasmusmc.nl

References

[1] Celsus A. De Medicina, with an English Translation by W. G. Spencer. 3 Vols. Cambridge: Harvard University Press; 1935-38

[2] Christopoulou-Aletra H, Papavramidou N. "Empyemas" of the thoracic cavity in the Hippocratic corpus. The Annals of Thoracic Surgery. 2008;**85**(3):1132-1134

[3] Walcott-Sapp S. The History of Pulmonary Lobectomy: Two Phases of Innovation. CTSNet. 2016. Available from: https://www.ctsnet.org/article/history-pulmonary-lobectomy-two-phases-innovation

[4] Estlander JA. Résection des côtes dans l'empyèma chronique. Revista medico-chirurgicala a Societatii de Medici si Naturalisti din Iasi (Paris). 1879;**3**:157-170

[5] Lister J. On the antiseptic principle in the practice of surgery. The Lancet. 1867;**90**(2299):353-356

[6] Barton M. The History of Surgical Gloves. 2018. Available from: https://www.pastmedicalhistory.co.uk/the-history-of-surgical-gloves/

[7] Hage JJ, Brinkman RJ. Andreas Vesalius' understanding of pulmonary ventilation. Respiratory Physiology & Neurobiology. 2016;**231**:37-44

[8] Sauerbruch F. Intrathoracic operations. Lancet. 1904;**7**:1308

[9] Meltzer A. Dr. Samuel James Meltzer and intratracheal anesthesia. 1990;**2**(1):54-58

[10] Meltzer SJ. Continuous respiration without respiratory movements. The Journal of Experimental Medicine. 1909;**11**(4):622-625

[11] Blum A. Alton ochsner, MD, 1896-1981 anti-smoking pioneer. The Ochsner Journal. 1999;**1**:102-105

[12] Ochsner A, Blalock J, Sucre A. Carcinoma of the stomach. The American Surgeon. 1955;**21**:1-16

[13] Churchill ED. The surgical treatment of carcinoma of the lung. The Journal of Thoracic Surgery. 1933;**2**:254-261

[14] Graham EA, Singer JJ. Successful removal of an entire lung for carcinoma of the bronchus. JAMA. 1984;**251**(2):257-260

[15] Ochsner A, DeBakey M. Primary pulmonary malignancy: Treatment by total pneumonectomy; analysis of 79 collected cases and presentation of 7 personal cases. The Ochsner Journal. 1999;**1**(3):109-125

[16] Shimkin MB, Connelly RR, Marcus SC, Cutler SJ. Pneumonectomy and lobectomy in bronchogenic carcinoma. A comparison of end results of the Overholt and Ochsner clinics. The Journal of Thoracic and Cardiovascular Surgery. 1962;**44**:503-519

[17] Kent EM, Blades B. The anatomic approach to pulmonary resection. Annals of Surgery. 1942;**116**(5):782-794

[18] Thomas CP. Conservative resection of the bronchial tree. Journal of the Royal College of Surgeons of Edinburgh. 1956;**1**(3):169-186

[19] Johnston JB, Jones PH. The treatment of bronchial carcinoma by lobectomy and sleeve resection of the main bronchus. Thorax. 1959;**14**(48):48-54

[20] Carlens E. Mediastinoscopy: A method for inspection and tissue biopsy in the superior mediastinum. Diseases of the Chest. 1959;**36**:343-352

[21] Kirklin JW, McDonald JR, Clagett OT, Moersch HJ, Gage RP.

Bronchogenic carcinoma: Cell type and other factors relating to prognosis. Surgery, Gynecology & Obstetrics. 1955;**100**(4):429-438

[22] Reynders H. Radicale' of 'conservatieve' pneumonectomie? Nederlands Tijdschrift voor Geneeskunde. 1962;**2257**

[23] Pearson FG, DeLarue NC, Ilves R, Todd TR, Cooper JD. Significance of positive superior mediastinal nodes identified at mediastinoscopy in patients with resectable cancer of the lung. The Journal of Thoracic and Cardiovascular Surgery. 1982;**83**(1):1-11

[24] Hoksch B, Birken-Bertsch H, Müller JM. Thoracoscopy before Jacobaeus. The Annals of Thoracic Surgery. 2002;**74**(4):1288-1290

[25] Lewis RJ, Caccavale RJ, Sisler GE. Imaged thorascopic surgery: A new thoracic technique for resection of mediastinal cysts. The Annals of Thoracic Surgery. 1992;**53**:38-20

[26] McKenna RJ Jr. Lobectomy by video-assisted thoracic surgery with mediastinal node sampling for lung cancer. The Journal of Thoracic and Cardiovascular Surgery. 1994;**107**(3):879-882

[27] Lim E. In hospital clinical efficacy, safety and oncologic outcomes from VIOLET: A UK multi-centre RCT of VATS versus open loebctomy for lung cancer. In: World Conference on Lung Cancer. London: Royal Brompton Hospital; 2019

[28] Bayman EO, Parekh KR, Keech J, Selte A, Brennan TJ. A prospective study of chronic pain after thoracic surgery. Anesthesiology. 2017;**126**(5):938-951

[29] Rocco G, Martin-Ucar A, Passera E. Uniportal VATS wedge pulmonary resections. The Annals of Thoracic Surgery. 2004;**77**(2):726-728

[30] Liu CC, Shih CS, Liu YH, Cheng CT, Melis E, Liu ZY. Subxiphoid single-port video-assisted thoracoscopic surgery. Journal of Visceral Surgery. 2016;**2**:112

[31] Zieliński M, Rami-Porta R. The Transcervical Approach in Thoracic Surgery. Berlin Heidelberg: Springer-Verlag; 2014. 221 p

[32] ElSaegh MMM, Ismail NA, Mydin MI, Nardini M, Dunning J. Subxiphoid uniportal lobectomy. Journal of Visceral Surgery. 2017;**3**:24

[33] Melfi F. Early experience with robotic technology for thoracoscopic surgery. European Journal of Cardio-Thoracic Surgery. 2002;**21**(5):864-868

[34] Subramanian MP, Colditz GA. Time trends of perioperative outcomes in early-stage non-small cell lung cancer resection patients (statistical commentary). Annals of Thoracic Surgery. 2019. Available online 19 October 2019. https://doi.org/10.1016/j.athoracsur.2019.09.031. In Press

[35] Aberle J, Reining F, Dannheim V, Flitsch J, Klinge A, Mann O. Metformin after bariatric surgery—An acid problem. Experimental and Clinical Endocrinology & Diabetes. 2012;**120**(3):152-153

[36] De Koning H, Van Der Aalst C, Ten Haaf K, Oudkerk M. PL02.05 effects of volume CT lung cancer screening: Mortality results of the NELSON randomised-controlled population based trial. Journal of Thoracic Oncology. 2018;**13**(10):S185

[37] Seguin-Givelet A, Grigoroiu M, Brian E, Gossot D. Planning and marking for thoracoscopic anatomical segmentectomies. Journal of Thoracic Disease. 2019;**10**:1187-1194

[38] Oizumi H, Kanauchi N, Kato H, Endoh M, Suzuki J, Fukaya K, et al. Anatomic thoracoscopic pulmonary

segmentectomy under 3-dimensional multidetector computed tomography simulation: A report of 52 consecutive cases. The Journal of Thoracic and Cardiovascular Surgery. 2011;**141**(3):678-682

[39] Saji H, Inoue T, Kato Y, Shimada Y, Hagiwara M, Kudo Y, et al. Virtual segmentectomy based on high-quality three-dimensional lung modelling from computed tomography images. Interactive Cardiovascular and Thoracic Surgery. 2013;**17**(2):227-232

[40] Shimizu K, Nakazawa S, Nagashima T, Kuwano H, Mogi A. 3D-CT anatomy for VATS segmentectomy. Journal of Visceral Surgery. 2017;**3**:88

[41] Wu WB, Xu XF, Wen W, Xu J, Zhu Q, Pan XL, et al. Three-dimensional computed tomography bronchography and angiography in the preoperative evaluation of thoracoscopic segmentectomy and subsegmentectomy. Journal of Thoracic Disease. 2016;**8**(Suppl 9):S710-S7S5

[42] Xue L, Fan H, Shi W, Ge D, Zhang Y, Wang Q, et al. Preoperative 3-dimensional computed tomography lung simulation before video-assisted thoracoscopic anatomic segmentectomy for ground glass opacity in lung. Journal of Thoracic Disease. 2018;**10**(12):6598-6605

[43] Chen-Yoshikawa TF, Date H. Update on three-dimensional image reconstruction for preoperative simulation in thoracic surgery. Journal of Thoracic Disease. 2016;**8**(Suppl 3): S295-S301

[44] Iwano S, Yokoi K, Taniguchi T, Kawaguchi K, Fukui T, Naganawa S. Planning of segmentectomy using three-dimensional computed tomography angiography with a virtual safety margin: Technique and initial experience. Lung Cancer. 2013;**81**(3):410-415

[45] Chinnock C. Virtual reality in surgery and medicine. Hospital Technology Series. 1994;**13**(18):1-48

[46] Shuhaiber JH. Augmented reality in surgery. Archives of Surgery. 2004;**139**(2):170-174

[47] Chytas D, Malahias MA, Nikolaou VS. Augmented reality in orthopedics: Current state and future directions. Frontiers in Surgery. 2019;**6**:38

[48] Guha D, Alotaibi NM, Nguyen N, Gupta S, McFaul C, Yang VXD. Augmented reality in neurosurgery: A review of current concepts and emerging applications. The Canadian Journal of Neurological Sciences. 2017;**44**(3):235-245

[49] Incekara F, Smits M, Dirven C, Vincent A. Clinical feasibility of a wearable mixed-reality device in neurosurgery. World Neurosurgery. 2018;**118**:e422-e427

[50] Shirk JD, Thiel DD, Wallen EM, Linehan JM, White WM, Badani KK, et al. Effect of 3-dimensional virtual reality models for surgical planning of robotic-assisted partial nephrectomy on surgical outcomes: A randomized clinical trial. JAMA Network Open. 2019;**2**(9):e1911598

[51] Tang R, Ma LF, Rong ZX, Li MD, Zeng JP, Wang XD, et al. Augmented reality technology for preoperative planning and intraoperative navigation during hepatobiliary surgery: A review of current methods. Hepatobiliary & Pancreatic Diseases International. 2018;**17**(2):101-112

[52] Jensen K, Bjerrum F, Hansen HJ, Petersen RH, Pedersen JH, Konge L. A new possibility in thoracoscopic virtual reality simulation training:

Development and testing of a novel virtual reality simulator for video-assisted thoracoscopic surgery lobectomy. Interactive Cardiovascular and Thoracic Surgery. 2015;**21**(4):420-426

[53] Frajhof L, Borges J, Hoffmann E, Lopes J, Haddad R. Virtual reality, mixed reality and augmented reality in surgical planning for video or robotically assisted thoracoscopic anatomic resections for treatment of lung cancer. Journal of Visualized Surgery. 2018;**4**:143

[54] Rouze S, de Latour B, Flecher E, Guihaire J, Castro M, Corre R, et al. Small pulmonary nodule localization with cone beam computed tomography during video-assisted thoracic surgery: A feasibility study. Interactive Cardiovascular and Thoracic Surgery. 2016;**22**(6):705-711

[55] Tan W, Ge W, Hang Y, Wu S, Liu S, Liu M. Computer assisted system for precise lung surgery based on medical image computing and mixed reality. Health Information Science and Systems. 2018;**6**(1):10

[56] Finkelstein SES, M R, Nguyen DM, Stewart JH, Tretler JA, Schrump DS. Virtual bronchoscopy for evaluation of malignant tumors of the thorax. The Journal of Thoracic and Cardiovascular Surgery. 2001;**123**(5):967-972

[57] Rapp-Bernhardt U, Welte T, Doehring W, Kropf S, Bernhardt TM. Diagnostic potential of virtual bronchoscopy: Advantages in comparison with axial CT slices, MPR and mIP? European Radiology. 2000;**10**(6):981-988

[58] Rossi S, Di Stasi M, Buscarini E, Cavanna L, Quaretti P, Squassante E, et al. Percutaneous radiofrequency interstitial thermal ablation in the treatment of small hepatocellular carcinoma. The Cancer Journal from Scientific American. 1995;**1**(1):73-81

[59] Shiina S, Teratani T, Obi S, Hamamura K, Koike Y, Omata M. Nonsurgical treatment of hepatocellular carcinoma: From percutaneous ethanol injection therapy and percutaneous microwave coagulation therapy to radiofrequency ablation. Oncology. 2002;**62**(Suppl 1):64-68

[60] Dupuy DE, DiPetrillo T, Gandhi S, Ready N, Ng T, Donat W, et al. Radiofrequency ablation followed by conventional radiotherapy for medically inoperable stage I non-small cell lung cancer. Chest. 2006;**129**(3):738-745

[61] Okuma T, Matsuoka T, Yamamoto A, Oyama Y, Hamamoto S, Toyoshima M, et al. Determinants of local progression after computed tomography-guided percutaneous radiofrequency ablation for unresectable lung tumors: 9-year experience in a single institution. Cardiovascular and Interventional Radiology. 2010;**33**(4):787-793

[62] Powell JW, Dexter E, Scalzetti EM, Bogart JA. Treatment advances for medically inoperable non-small-cell lung cancer: Emphasis on prospective trials. The Lancet Oncology. 2009;**10**(9):885-894

[63] Gillams A. Ablation of lung tumours. Cancer Imaging. 2012;**12**:361-362

[64] Hiraki T, Gobara H, Iishi T, Sano Y, Iguchi T, Fujiwara H, et al. Percutaneous radiofrequency ablation for clinical stage I non-small cell lung cancer: Results in 20 nonsurgical candidates. The Journal of Thoracic and Cardiovascular Surgery. 2007;**134**(5):1306-1312

[65] Pennathur A, Luketich JD, Abbas G, Chen M, Fernando HC, Gooding WE, et al. Radiofrequency ablation for the

treatment of stage I non-small cell lung cancer in high-risk patients. The Journal of Thoracic and Cardiovascular Surgery. 2007;**134**(4):857-864

[66] Simon CJ, Dupuy DE, DiPetrillo TA, Safran HP, Grieco CA, Ng T, et al. Pulmonary radiofrequency ablation: Long-term safety and efficacy in 153 patients. Radiology. 2007;**243**(1):268-275

[67] Thanos L, Mylona S, Pomoni M, Athanassiadi K, Theakos N, Zoganas L, et al. Percutaneous radiofrequency thermal ablation of primary and metastatic lung tumors. European Journal of Cardio-Thoracic Surgery. 2006;**30**(5):797-800

[68] Dupuy DE, Fernando HC, Hillman S, Ng T, Tan AD, Sharma A, et al. Radiofrequency ablation of stage IA non-small cell lung cancer in medically inoperable patients: Results from the American College of Surgeons Oncology Group Z4033 (Alliance) trial. Cancer. 2015;**121**(19):3491-3498

[69] Hiraki T, Gobara H, Mimura H, Matsui Y, Toyooka S, Kanazawa S. Percutaneous radiofrequency ablation of clinical stage I non-small cell lung cancer. The Journal of Thoracic and Cardiovascular Surgery. 2011;**142**(1):24-30

[70] Liu B, Liu L, Hu M, Qian K, Li Y. Percutaneous radiofrequency ablation for medically inoperable patients with clinical stage I non-small cell lung cancer. Thoracic Cancer. 2015;**6**(3):327-333

[71] Ambrogi MC, Fanucchi O, Cioni R, Dini P, De Liperi A, Cappelli C, et al. Long-term results of radiofrequency ablation treatment of stage I non-small cell lung cancer: A prospective intention-to-treat study. Journal of Thoracic Oncology. 2011;**6**(12):2044-2051

[72] Palussiere J, Marcet B, Descat E, Deschamps F, Rao P, Ravaud A, et al. Lung tumors treated with percutaneous radiofrequency ablation: Computed tomography imaging follow-up. Cardiovascular and Interventional Radiology. 2011;**34**(5):989-997

[73] Simon TG, Beland MD, Machan JT, Dipetrillo T, Dupuy DE. Charlson comorbidity index predicts patient outcome, in cases of inoperable non-small cell lung cancer treated with radiofrequency ablation. European Journal of Radiology. 2012;**81**(12):4167-4172

[74] Li G, Xue M, Chen W, Yi S. Efficacy and safety of radiofrequency ablation for lung cancers: A systematic review and meta-analysis. European Journal of Radiology. 2018;**100**:92-98

[75] Yuan Z, Wang Y, Zhang J, Zheng J, Li WA. Meta-analysis of clinical outcomes after radiofrequency ablation and microwave ablation for lung cancer and pulmonary metastases. Journal of the American College of Radiology. 2019;**16**(3)

[76] Dupuy DE, Zagoria RJ, Akerley W, Mayo-Smith WW, Kavanagh PV, Safran H. Percutaneous radiofrequency ablation of malignancies in the lung. AJR. American Journal of Roentgenology. 2000;**174**(1):57-59

[77] Robert Sheu Y, Hong K. Percutaneous lung tumor ablation. Techniques in Vascular and Interventional Radiology. 2013;**16**(4):239-252

[78] Mouli SK, Kurilova I, Sofocleous CT, Lewandowski RJ. The role of percutaneous image-guided thermal ablation for the treatment of pulmonary malignancies. AJR. American Journal of Roentgenology. 2017;**209**(4):740-751

[79] Gage AA, Baust J. Mechanisms of tissue injury in cryosurgery. Cryobiology. 1998;**37**(3):171-186

[80] Niu L, Xu K, Mu F. Cryosurgery for lung cancer. Journal of Thoracic Disease. 2012;**4**(4):408-419

[81] McDevitt JL, Mouli SK, Nemcek AA, Lewandowski RJ, Salem R, Sato KT. Percutaneous cryoablation for the treatment of primary and metastatic lung tumors: Identification of risk factors for recurrence and major complications. Journal of Vascular and Interventional Radiology. 2016;**27**(9):1371-1379

[82] Moore W, Talati R, Bhattacharji P, Bilfinger T. Five-year survival after cryoablation of stage I non-small cell lung cancer in medically inoperable patients. Journal of Vascular and Interventional Radiology. 2015;**26**(3):312-319

[83] Uhlig J, Case MD, Blasberg JD, Boffa DJ, Chiang A, Gettinger SN, et al. Comparison of survival rates after a combination of local treatment and systemic therapy vs systemic therapy alone for treatment of stage IV non-small cell lung cancer. JAMA Network Open. 2019;**2**(8):e199702

[84] Yamauchi Y, Izumi Y, Hashimoto K, Yashiro H, Inoue M, Nakatsuka S, et al. Percutaneous cryoablation for the treatment of medically inoperable stage I non-small cell lung cancer. PLoS One. 2012;**7**(3):e33223

[85] Yamauchi Y, Izumi Y, Kawamura M, Nakatsuka S, Yashiro H, Tsukada N, et al. Percutaneous cryoablation of pulmonary metastases from colorectal cancer. PLoS One. 2011;**6**(11):e27086

[86] Maiwand MO, Asimakopoulos G. Cryosurgery for lung cancer: Clinical results and technical aspects. Technology in Cancer Research & Treatment. 2004;**3**(2):143-150

Chapter 9

Advances in Minimally Invasive Surgery for Lung Cancer

Rachit Shah and Nils-Tomas Delagar McBride

Abstract

Over the last 25 years, improvement in instrumentation and surgical techniques has led to widespread adaptation of thoracoscopic (VATS) surgery in the field of thoracic oncology. What once was a niche operation like VATS wedge resection to now hybrid VATS chest wall resections, and advanced surgeries like bronchoplasty and sleeve resections are done with VATS. This has led to improved surgical outcomes for our patients and increased use of surgery in the treatment of chest disease. We review the history of VATS and its current state with most recent changes and upgrades in the technique in this chapter. We review the advancement in uniportal VATS, robotic assisted resection, complex VATS resection, and awake lung surgery with VATS.

Keywords: VATS, uniportal, robotics, awake VATS, hybrid resections

1. History of thoracoscopy

While the modern era of thoracoscopy begins in the early 1990s and includes Giancarlo Roviaro's report of the first thoracoscopic lobectomy as a major milestone [1], the term thoracoscopy dates back to a procedure performed by Francis Richard Cruise and Samuel Gordon in 1865 [2]. Using a device similar to the "Leichtleiter" used by Bozzini with a light source improved by Antonin Jean Desormeaux, Cruise examined the pleural space of an 11 years old suffering from an empyema and a pleurocutaneous fistula. Several years later, in 1882, coincidentally the year Robert Koch discovered *Mycobacterium tuberculosis* [3], Carlo Forlanini observed that spontaneous pneumothorax could collapse cavitary lesions and lead to their resolution [4]. From this observation, he introduced a procedure of inducing artificial closed pneumothoraces by inserting a needle in the anterior axillary line and forcing air into the pleural space, the first minimally invasive thoracic procedure.

Though he is considered by many to be the father of thoracoscopy, Hans Christian Jacobeus published his eponymous Jacobeus Operation in 1910; this operation involved inducing pneumothorax, inserting a thoracoscope through one incision, and introducing an galvanocautery instrument in through a separate incision for the purpose of releasing adhesions to allow the lung collapse to treat pulmonary tuberculosis [5]. Subsequently, antibiotics, improved anesthetics, and intraoperative oxygen delivery, thoracoscopy was neglected as a therapeutic option for most of the twentieth century until the modern era.

Attributed in large part to fiber optics for light transmission, enhanced image processing and rendering, and the advent of the surgical staplers, interest in VATS was piqued. The classic three-port technique focused the camera from hip-to-head while increased experience determined that a modified approach should focus from umbilicus-to-shoulder. Aside from traditional three-port VATS technique, some procedures, including thoracic sympathectomy, have been performed via needlescopic VATS as well as two-port and uniportal VATS. Additionally, robotic assisted thoracic surgery (RATS) can serve a role in thoracic surgery, particularly for mediastinal procedures. Each of these different techniques has the potential to serve an important role as part of the thoracic surgeon's armamentarium [6].

2. VATS lobectomy

As mentioned in the previous section, Roviaro reported the first VATS lobectomy in 1991. However, in 1993, only 2% of the cases reported by the Video Assisted Study Group were VATS lobectomies while 49% were wedge resections. As reports continued to show the feasibility of VATS lobectomies as well as possible advantages, familiarity with the procedure improved technique. Even so, skepticism remained for the use of VATS for the treatment of non-small cell lung cancer (NSCLC). The results of a randomized control trial by Kirby et al. [7] failed to demonstrate the superiority of VATS though it also failed to demonstrate inferiority. In this study, 30 patients were randomized to the traditional muscle-sparing thoracotomy while 24 were put into the VATS group. No difference was found between the duration of chest tube drainage, hospital length of stay, pain score, or time prior to returning to work. The study specifically expressed concerns about the adequacy of lymph node dissection for an operation intended for malignancy.

McKenna et al. reviewed 298 cases of patients that underwent VATS lobectomy and lymph node dissection for NSCLC with the intent of determining adequacy of resection [8]. Their multi-institutional review included patients with stage I to IIIA and featured a 6% conversion rate with a single report of an incisional recurrence. In this study, the survival rate at 4 years for patients with stage I disease was 70%. Comparatively, Li and Wang [9] retrospectively evaluated outcomes for 76 patients that underwent lobectomies with lymph node dissection via VATS or thoracotomy for clinical N0 disease that was discovered to be pathologic N2 NSCLC. In their study, the number of lymph nodes recovered and the number of stations sampled were similar. The survival and disease-free survival rates are presented in **Table 1**. In addition to these reported survival and disease-free survival rates, VATS patients had shorter operative times and less blood loss.

A subsequent larger study was performed by Onaitis et al. [10] on VATS lobectomies for benign and malignant disease including 500 patients. Of these lobectomies, 83.2% were performed for NSCLC with an overall conversion rate of 1.6% (8 of 500). The pathologic stage of the patients included in this study were stage I (55.3%), stage II (9.6%) and stage III or greater (10.6%). The overall 2-year survival rate in the patients with stage I NSCLC and stage II was comparable to those undergoing thoracotomy (85% vs. 77%). Additionally, perioperative mortality for benign pathologies was 0% while it was 1% for malignant pathologies.

	1-year disease-free survival	3-year disease-free survival	1-year survival	3-year survival
VATS	82.6%	49.3%	84.9%	64.0%
Thoracotomy	72.0%	51.3%	71.2%	42.7%

Table 1.
Comparative survival rates.

Whitson et al. [11] analyzed 147 patients who underwent lobectomies for stage I NSCLC (59 by VATS and 88 by thoracotomy). In this particular study, patients who underwent thoracotomy had a larger yield of nodes and shorter time in the ICU, potentially because of the additional comorbidities reported in the VATS patients. However, no significant differences were found in operative times, length of hospital stay, or median survival.

3. Long-term outcomes of VATS lobectomy for NSCLC

To justify the continued use of VATS for lobectomies as treatment for NSCLC, data continues to be collected and reported by many groups. Multi-institutional experience of 145 patients with clinical stage IA NSCLC less than or equal to 2 cm was reported by Shigemura et al. [12]. For this study, three approaches were utilized: complete thoracoscopic technique without any rib spreading, assisted VATS, which included VATS with a mini-thoracotomy and open thoractomy. The overall 5-year survival rates did not differ significantly between techniques (VATS—96.7%, assisted VATS—95.2%, and open—97.2%). Higuchi et al. [13] also reported their experience of 160 patients with stage IA NSCLC with patients who underwent VATS lobectomy and open thoracotomy. The reported 5-year disease-free survival was equivalent with 88% in the VATS group and 77.1% in the thoracotomy group. The 5-year overall survival for pathologic stage IA NSCLC was 94.8% in the VATS group and 96.2% in the thoracotomy group, showing no statistical difference in survival. Lee et al. [14] performed a retrospective review of patients who underwent lobectomy for NSCLC, from their institution using propensity-matched scores in 416 patients. The review included clinical stage I to III with the majority being stage IA. The 3- and 5-year overall survival for the patients with clinical stage IA who underwent VATS lobectomy were 87.4 and 76.5%, respectively, and 81.6 and 77.5% for thoracotomy. Their analysis also showed no inferiority of VATS lobectomy for early stage NSCLC. Murakawa et al. [15] also evaluated survival outcomes in patients with early stage NSCLC and found VATS and open thoracotomy to be equivalent. Yang et al. [16] queried the national cancer database to evaluate the national survival outcomes following VATS versus open lobectomy for stage I NSCLC. After propensity score matching 2928 patients were included in the final analysis. In the matched patients there was no difference in 5-year survival between VATS and open thoracotomy, 66.3 and 65.8%, respectively. Data published by Flores et al. [17], which included intent to treat analysis in 741 patients (398 VATS and 343 open thoracotomy) demonstrating similar 5 year survival. The majority of their patients treated with lobectomy were clinical stage IA and demonstrated 79% 5-year survival in the VATS group and 75% in the open thoracotomy group (**Table 2**).

Reference	Year	# of patients	VATS	Open
Shigemura et al. [12]	2006	145	96.7%	97.2%
Flores et al. [17]	2009	741	79%	75%
Higuchi et al. [13]	2014	160	94.8%	96.2%
Lee et al. [14]	2013	416	76.5%	77.5%
Yang et al. [18]	2017	2928	66.3%	65.8%

Table 2.
Five-year overall survival.

4. Mediastinal lymph node dissection (MLND) via VATS

An essential component of each complete pulmonary resection for NSCLC is an adequate mediastinal lymph node dissection (MLND). With the advent of VATS lobectomy particularly for NSCLC, the efficacy of a VATS MLND has been evaluated in comparison to MLND via thoracotomy. The National Comprehensive Cancer Network's (NCCN) NSCLC Database was evaluated by D'Amico et al. [19] to compare VATS MLND to MLND via thoracotomy. The number of lymph node stations evaluated by both techniques was at least 3 and the number of N2 nodes evaluated by both techniques was not significantly different. A single institution randomized control trial reported by Palade et al. [20] included 66 patients with stage 1 NSCLC. In this study, there was no statistically significant difference in the overall number of lymph nodes sampled or the number of lymph nodes in each station. Because VATS MLND has comparable efficacy to open dissection, adequate lymph node dissection can be performed thoracoscopically.

5. Clinical advantages of VATS lobectomy vs. thoracotomy

Multiple studies have documented several advantages of VATS lobectomies including improved quality of life, decreased postoperative pain, and shorter hospital stays. A retrospective study by Villazmizar et al. [21] evaluated 1097 patients that underwent lobectomies with 697 lobectomies via VATS and 382 lobectomies via thoracotomy. In reviewing these cases, the incidence of postoperative complications, including atrial fibrillation, atelectasis, prolonged air leak, transfusion requirements, pneumonia, renal failure death, and shorter hospital stay, were all found to be less common in the VATS lobectomy group. Paul et al. [22] found similar results in evaluating the STS database and reviewing 6323 lobectomies, 5024 via thoracotomy and 1281 via VATS. Propensity matched analysis of these cases found that 73% of VATS patients experienced no complications while 65.3% of thoracotomy patients had no complications. Furthermore, patients undergoing VATS lobectomy in this review had a lower incidence of arrhythmias, reintubations, and blood transfusion as well as shorter duration of chest tube drainage and length of stay.

Predictably, patients requiring pulmonary resections for management of NSCLC often suffer from decreased pulmonary function, which makes them high risk. Because VATS has reduced the risks associated with lobectomy, patients previously considered prohibitive risks are potentially resectable. Donahoe et al. [23] evaluated a cohort of 608 patients (including 72 high risk and 536 standard risk) that underwent lobectomy for NSCLC. For those patients who underwent a VATS lobectomy, there was no difference in complication rate or overall survival between high risk and standard risk patients. Another study by Bertani et al. [24] found that VATS lobectomy patients with reduced preoperative FEV1 had similar outcomes as those with normal preoperative FEV1, despite a longer hospital stay. Patient with a predicted postoperative FEV1% of less than 60% had an average length of stay of 8.7 days while those with a predicted postoperative FEV1% of greater than 60% was 6.8 days (8.7 vs. 6.8 days, $p = 0.05$) (**Table 3**).

In light of these advantages, it is important to establish not only efficacy but cost effectiveness as a measure of quality. Swanson et al. [25] evaluated the costs of open versus VATS lobectomy for 3961. In this study, patients who underwent a VATS lobectomy had a shorter length of stay, less adverse events, and cost the hospital less than an open lobectomy.

Ppo FEV1%	n	Grade I	Grade II	Grade IIIa	Grade IIIb	p-value†	LOS, Mean (±SD)	p-value‡
<40%	2	0 (—)	1 (100.00)	0 (—)	0 (—)	n.s	5.90 (±2.23)	n.s
≥40%	98	22 (45.83)	24 (50.00)	1 (2.08)	1 (2.08)		7.18 (±3.83)	
<50%	4	1 (50.00)	1 (50.00)	0 (—)	0 (—)	n.s	9.18 (±6.31)	n.s
≥50%	96	21 (44.68)	24 (51.06)	1 (2.13)	1 (2.13)		7.10 (±3.72)	
<60%	18	4 (40.00)	4 (40.00)	1 (10.00)	1 (10.00)	0.067	8.74 (±4.79)	0.05
≥60%	82	18 (46.15)	21 (53.85)	0 (—)	0 (—)		6.80 (±3.52)	

LOS, overall hospital length of stay; n.s., not significant; ppo-FEV1, predicted postoperative forced expiratory volume in 1 s; SD, standard deviation.
†Fisher's exact test.
‡t-test with equal or unequal variance.

Table 3.
Complications of patients undergoing video-assisted thoracic surgery lobectomy based on different ppo-FEV1 cut-offs [24].

6. Clinical advantages of VATS lobectomy vs. thoracotomy

As a direct result of the advantages and similar survival rates for patients after VATS lobectomy for NSCLC, many institutions have adopted this surgical approach. In addition to VATS lobectomies, other anatomic resections have been performed via VATS.

Recent data have indicated that an anatomic segmentectomy can be considered an acceptable operation to obtain an R0 resection for small stage I NSCLC lesions. In a study reviewing 225 anatomic segmentectomies by Schuchert et al. [26], VATS segmentectomies were compared to those performed via thoracotomy demonstrating similar overall mortality, complications, recurrence rates, and overall survival.

Liu et al. [27] difference was seen in transfusion rates, number of lymph nodes dissected, estimated blood loss, duration of chest tube drainage, overall complication rates, or length of hospital stay. Operative time was longer in the VATS group while postoperative mean pain scores were higher in the higher in the thoracotomy group. From their data, they conclude that VATS pneumonectomy is a safe technique for either benign or malignant disease.

7. Development of single port VATS

The first description of single port VATS by Rocco et al. [28] was published in 2004. Initially used for diagnosis or treatment of primary spontaneous pneumothorax, the uses of single port VATS expanded to include management of pleural effusions, nonanatomic wedge resections, and diagnostic thoracoscopy for lung cancer during this study's 10 year experience. The conversion rate to a 2 or 3 port VATS or mini thoracotomy was 3.7%. Xie et al. [29] reported their single-institution experience of single port VATS in 1063 cases with a conversion rate of 4.6%. Institutional data reported by Shih et al. [30] comparing single port VATS to multiport VATS for anatomic segmentectomies in treating primary lung cancer indicated similar operative outcomes in the two propensity matched groups.

Single port VATS has been evaluated for safety and efficacy in the treatment of NSCLC. Comparing VATS and single port VATS lobectomy patients, Dai et al. [31] reported that single port VATS patients reported a higher satisfaction score, less postoperative pain, and less blood loss. Fan et al. [32] reported a similar operative time and number of lymph nodes dissected in both single port VATS and open lobectomies for locally advanced NSCLC. In this study, single port patients had a shorter period of chest tube drainage and length of hospital stay but a higher complication rate than thoracotomy. The complications studied included prolonged air leak, atrial fibrillation, bleeding, pneumonia, bronchopleural fistula, chylothorax, death, and 30-day mortality. However, neither study reported data on recurrence rates of overall survival.

8. Development of robotic-assisted VATS

With data indicating that VATS is safe and efficacious for the resection of NSCLC as well as having a variety of advantages over open surgery, it has been established as the preferred technique. However, with the availability of the robotic assistance, techniques for robotic procedures have been developed and examined. Utilizing three robotic ports as well as an assistance port, Melfi et al. [33] reported their early experience using the Da Vinci platform, describing lobectomies, enucleations, excisions, and bulla stitching. Single institution experiences have reported safety and shown similar outcomes in robotic resection when compared to VATS with improvement in postoperative pain. Other experiences with larger cohorts found higher incidence of operative injury, and bleeding compared to VATS. Robotic-assisted operations are also significantly more costly [34]. Park et al. [35] reported the long-term oncologic outcomes from three institutions and found them to be similar to VATS lobectomies.

Rajaram et al. [36] evaluated the use of robotic surgery for stage I to IIa NSCLC in the National Cancer Database from 2010 to 2012. They found 62,206 patients who underwent lobectomies including the open (n = 45,427), VATS (n = 12,990), and robotic (n = 3689) techniques. They found that the over the two-year period the use of the robotic lobectomy technique increased by 6%. Patients who underwent a robotic lobectomy had a lower length of stay compared to open lobectomy but had a higher rate of prolonged length of stay compared to VATS. The number of lymph nodes examined was significantly higher in the VATS group compared to robotic, with no difference in number of lymph nodes in the robotic and open groups. The resection status, margin positivity, was comparable between all groups. The evaluation of this data and the known increase in cost for the robotic technique did not show any potential advantages to the use of robotic surgery for a lobectomy compared to VATS. With the use of robotic techniques in treatment for NSCLC, early outcomes have been evaluated. Mungo et al. [37] found no negative effect on outcomes in patients who underwent robotic resection.

Park et al. [38] reported long-term outcomes to be similar in robotic assisted lobectomies compared to VATS and open thoracotomy. Yang et al. [18] compared the use of robotic, VATS, and open thoracotomy in patients treated with lobectomy for stage I NSCLC. An advantage of the robotic approach they report is a higher number of mediastinal lymph node stations dissected compared to the other techniques. The patients treated with the minimally invasive approach, robotic and VATS, had shorter hospital stays. The long term outcomes were similar in all the groups with 5 year overall survival reported for robotic, VATS and open thoracotomy as 77.6%, 73.5%, and 77.9%, respectively.

Cerfolio et al. [39] demonstrated the efficacy of robotic segmentectomies. For 100 planned robotic segmentectomies, 7 converted to lobectomies though every case was completed robotically. In this cohort, there were no mortalities at 30 or 90 days. Only 2 patients suffered major morbidity, each of which were postoperative pneumonias. Of the 79 patients that underwent robotic segmentectomy, there were only 3 recurrences (3.4%) with median follow up of 30 months while overall survival was 95%.

9. Development of awake VATS

Optimal visualization for a VATS is typically achieved with general anesthesia for double lumen tube intubation. However, awake VATS under regional anesthesia may be appropriate for selected patients. Potential anesthetic approaches include intercostal nerve block, paravertebral block, thoracic epidural block, peripheral field block, or ipsilateral stellate ganglion block [40].

A randomized study of 43 patients by Pompeo et al. [41] assessed the feasibility and efficacy of awake VATS in patients with spontaneous pneumothoraces that require intervention. Patients were randomized to undergo VATS bullectomy and pleural abrasion with either thoracic epidural anesthesia or general anesthesia. The patients undergoing awake VATS had shorter operating room times, improved pain scores, and shorter hospital stays compared to the general anesthesia group. Awake VATS patients did suffer minor complications including vomiting and transient urinary retention though there was no difference in morbidity and mortality between groups. Recurrences at 12 months were similar in each group. Tacconi et al. [42] reported satisfactory lung reexpansion in 95% in 19 patients that underwent awake VATS for pleural decortication. A single institution study by Chen et al. [43] reported 285 cases of awake VATS for pathologies such as primary lung cancer, metastatic lung cancer, benign lung tumors, and pneumothorax. Operative interventions included lobectomies, wedge resections and segmentectomies with a 4.9% intubation rate.

Additionally, Chen et al. [44] examined outcomes for patient undergoing awake VATS in stage I and II NSCLC. For 30 patients undergoing awake VATS lobectomy under epidural anesthesia and intrathoracic vagal block with sedation and 30 patients undergoing VATS lobectomy under general anesthesia with single lung ventilation, there was evidence that each group had comparable pathologic stages and number of lymph nodes resected. Additionally, no statistical difference was seen in postoperative complication though the awake VATS group had shorter hospital stays and decreased need for chest tube drainage.

10. Conclusion

At this point in the development of minimally invasive thoracic surgery, there is evidence that there are advantages as well as proof of non-inferiority. Additionally, robotic-assisted minimally invasive surgery has been proven safe in the hands of those adept in it on selected patients but carries the burden of additional cost. Follow up data from some studies show that long term outcomes are equivalent. Additional study is still required to fully establish if the costs of robotic surgery are justified.

Author details

Rachit Shah* and Nils-Tomas Delagar McBride
Virginia Commonwealth University Medical Center, USA

*Address all correspondence to: rachit.shah@vcuhealth.org

References

[1] Roviaro GC, Rebuffat C, Varoli F, Vergani C, Mariani C, Maciocco M. Videoendoscopic pulmonary lobectomy for cancer. Surgical Laparoscopy & Endoscopy. 1992;**2**:244-247

[2] Gordon S. Clinical reports of rare cases, occurring in the Whitworth and Harwicke Hospitals. Dublin Quarterly Journal of Medical Science. 1866

[3] Koch R. "Die Aetiologie der Tuberculose" [The etiology of tuberculosis]. Berliner Klinische Wochenschrift (Berlin Clinical Weekly). 1882;**19**:221-230

[4] Forlanini C. A contribuzioni della terapia chirurgica della tisi-Ablazione del polmone? Pneumotorace artificiale? Gazz Osp. 1882;**3**(68):53729, 585-587, 601-602, 609-610, 617-619, 625-627, 641-643, 657-660, 665-667, 689-691, 705-707

[5] Jacobaeus H. Ueber die moglichkeit die zystoskopie bei untersuchung seroser Honlungen Munchen. Deutsche Medizinische Wchenschrift. 1910;**57**:2090-2092

[6] Sihoe AD. The evolution of minimally invasive thoracic surgery: Implications for the practice of uniportal thoracoscopic surgery. Journal of Thoracic Disease. 2014;**6**(Suppl 6): S604-S617. DOI: 10.3978/j.issn.2072-1439.2014.08.52

[7] Kirby TJ, Mack MJ, Landreneau RJ, Rice TW. Lobectomy–video-assisted thoracic surgery versus muscle-sparing thoracotomy. A randomized trial. The Journal of Thoracic and Cardiovascular Surgery. 1995;**109**(5):997-1001; discussion -2

[8] McKenna RJ Jr, Wolf RK, Brenner M, Fischel RJ, Wurnig P. Is lobectomy by video-assisted thoracic surgery an adequate cancer operation? The Annals of Thoracic Surgery. 1998;**66**(6):1903-1908

[9] Li Y, Wang J. Comparison of clinical outcomes for patients with clinical N0 and pathologic N2 non-small cell lung cancer after thoracoscopic lobectomy and open lobectomy: A retrospective analysis of 76 patients. Journal of Surgical Oncology. 2012;**106**(4):431-435

[10] Onaitis MW, Petersen RP, Balderson SS, Toloza E, Burfeind WR, Harpole DH Jr, et al. Thoracoscopic lobectomy is a safe and versatile procedure: Experience with 500 consecutive patients. Annals of Surgery. 2006;**244**(3):420-425

[11] Whitson BA, Andrade RS, Boettcher A, Bardales R, Kratzke RA, Dahlberg PS, et al. Video-assisted thoracoscopic surgery is more favorable than thoracotomy for resection of clinical stage I non-small cell lung cancer. The Annals of Thoracic Surgery. 2007;**83**(6):1965-1970

[12] Shigemura N, Akashi A, Funaki S, Nakagiri T, Inoue M, Sawabata N, et al. Long-term outcomes after a variety of video-assisted thoracoscopic lobectomy approaches for clinical stage IA lung cancer: A multi-institutional study. The Journal of thoracic and cardiovascular surgery. 2006;**132**(3):507-512

[13] Higuchi M, Yaginuma H, Yonechi A, Kanno R, Ohishi A, Suzuki H, et al. Long-term outcomes after video-assisted thoracic surgery (VATS) lobectomy versus lobectomy via open thoracotomy for clinical stage IA non-small cell lung cancer. Journal of Cardiothoracic Surgery. 2014;**9**:88

[14] Lee PC, Nasar A, Port JL, Paul S, Stiles B, Chiu YL, et al. Long-term survival after lobectomy for non-small cell lung cancer by video-assisted thoracic surgery versus thoracotomy.

The Annals of Thoracic Surgery. 2013;**96**(3):951-960; discussion 60-1

[15] Murakawa T, Ichinose J, Hino H, Kitano K, Konoeda C, Nakajima J. Long-term outcomes of open and video-assisted thoracoscopic lung lobectomy for the treatment of early stage non-small cell lung cancer are similar: A propensity-matched study. World Journal of Surgery. 2015;**39**(5):1084-1091

[16] Yang CF, Meyerhoff RR, Mayne NR, Singhapricha T, Toomey CB, Speicher PJ, et al. Long-term survival following open versus thoracoscopic lobectomy after preoperative chemotherapy for non-small cell lung cancer. European Journal of Cardio-thoracic Surgery: Official Journal of the European Association for Cardio-Thoracic Surgery. 2016;**49**(6):1615-1623

[17] Flores RM, Park BJ, Dycoco J, Aronova A, Hirth Y, Rizk NP, et al. Lobectomy by video-assisted thoracic surgery (VATS) versus thoracotomy for lung cancer. The Journal of Thoracic and Cardiovascular Surgery. 2009;**138**(1):11-18

[18] Yang HX, Woo KM, Sima CS, Bains MS, Adusumilli PS, Huang J, et al. Long-term survival based on the surgical approach to lobectomy for clinical stage I nonsmall cell lung Cancer: Comparison of robotic, video-assisted thoracic surgery, and thoracotomy lobectomy. Annals of Surgery. 2017;**265**(2):431-437

[19] D'Amico TA, Niland J, Mamet R, Zornosa C, Dexter EU, Onaitis MW. Efficacy of mediastinal lymph node dissection during lobectomy for lung cancer by thoracoscopy and thoracotomy. The Annals of Thoracic Surgery. 2011;**92**(1):226-231; Discussion 31-2

[20] Palade E, Passlick B, Osei-Agyemang T, Gunter J, Wiesemann S. Video-assisted vs open mediastinal lymphadenectomy for stage I non-small-cell lung cancer: Results of a prospective randomized trial. European Journal of Cardio-Thoracic Surgery: Official Journal of the European Association for Cardio-Thoracic Surgery. 2013;**44**(2):244-249; Discussion 9

[21] Villamizar NR, Darrabie MD, Burfeind WR, Petersen RP, Onaitis MW, Toloza E, et al. Thoracoscopic lobectomy is associated with lower morbidity compared with thoracotomy. The Journal of Thoracic and Cardiovascular Surgery. 2009;**138**(2):419-425

[22] Paul S, Altorki NK, Sheng S, Lee PC, Harpole DH, Onaitis MW, et al. Thoracoscopic lobectomy is associated with lower morbidity than open lobectomy: A propensity-matched analysis from the STS database. The Journal of Thoracic and Cardiovascular Surgery. 2010;**139**(2):366-378

[23] Donahoe LL, de Valence M, Atenafu EG, Hanna WC, Waddell TK, Pierre AF, et al. High risk for thoracotomy but not thoracoscopic lobectomy. The Annals of Thoracic Surgery. 2017

[24] Bertani A, Ferrari PA, De Monte L, Russo E, Di Paola G. Video-assisted thoracic surgery lobectomy in patients with reduced pulmonary function: A single-center series. Future Oncology (London, England). 2016;**12**(23s):39-45

[25] Swanson SJ, Meyers BF, Gunnarsson CL, Moore M, Howington JA, Maddaus MA, et al. Video-assisted thoracoscopic lobectomy is less costly and morbid than open lobectomy: A retrospective multiinstitutional database analysis. The Annals of Thoracic Surgery. 2012;**93**(4):1027-1032

[26] Schuchert MJ, Pettiford BL, Pennathur A, Abbas G, Awais O,

Close J, et al. Anatomic segmentectomy for stage I non-small-cell lung cancer: Comparison of video-assisted thoracic surgery versus open approach. The Journal of Thoracic and Cardiovascular Surgery. 2009;**138**(6):1318-25.e1

[27] Liu Y, Gao Y, Zhang H, Cheng Y, Chang R, Zhang W, et al. Video-assisted versus conventional thoracotomy pneumonectomy: A comparison of perioperative outcomes and short-term measures of convalescence. Journal of Thoracic Disease. 2016;**8**(12):3537-3542

[28] Rocco G, Martin-Ucar A, Passera E. Uniportal VATS wedge pulmonary resections. The Annals of Thoracic Surgery. 2004;**77**(2):726-728

[29] Xie D, Wang H, Fei K, Chen C, Zhao D, Zhou X, et al. Single-port video-assisted thoracic surgery in 1063 cases: A single-institution experiencedagger. European Journal of Cardio-Thoracic Surgery: Official Journal of the European Association for Cardio-thoracic Surgery. 2016;**49**(Suppl 1):i31-i36

[30] Shih CS, Liu CC, Liu ZY, Pennarun N, Cheng CT. Comparing the postoperative outcomes of video-assisted thoracoscopic surgery (VATS) segmentectomy using a multi-port technique versus a single-port technique for primary lung cancer. Journal of Thoracic Disease. 2016;**8**(Suppl 3): S287-S294

[31] Dai F, Meng S, Mei L, Guan C, Ma Z. Single-port video-assisted thoracic surgery in the treatment of non-small cell lung cancer: A propensity-matched comparative analysis. Journal of Thoracic Disease. 2016;**8**(10):2872-2878

[32] Fan J, Yao J, Wang Q, Chang Z. Safety and feasibility of uniportal video-assisted thoracoscopic surgery for locally advanced non-small cell lung cancer. Journal of Thoracic Disease. 2016;**8**(12):3543-3550

[33] Melfi FM, Menconi GF, Mariani AM, Angeletti CA. Early experience with robotic technology for thoracoscopic surgery. European Journal of Cardio-Thoracic Surgery: Official Journal of the European Association for Cardio-thoracic Surgery. 2002;**21**(5):864-868

[34] Park BJ, Flores RM. Cost comparison of robotic, video-assisted thoracic surgery and thoracotomy approaches to pulmonary lobectomy. Thoracic Surgery Clinics. 2008;**18**(3):297-300; vii

[35] Park BJ. Robotic lobectomy for non-small cell lung cancer: Long-term oncologic results. Thoracic Surgery Clinics. 2014;**24**(2):157-162; vi

[36] Rajaram R, Mohanty S, Bentrem DJ, Pavey ES, Odell DD, Bharat A, et al. Nationwide assessment of robotic lobectomy for non-small cell lung cancer. The Annals of Thoracic Surgery. 2017;**103**(4):1092-1100

[37] Mungo B, Hooker CM, Ho JS, Yang SC, Battafarano RJ, Brock MV, et al. Robotic versus thoracoscopic resection for lung cancer: Early results of a new robotic program. Journal of Laparoendoscopic & Advanced Surgical Techniques Part A. 2016;**26**(4):243-248

[38] Park BJ, Melfi F, Mussi A, Maisonneuve P, Spaggiari L, Da Silva RK, et al. Robotic lobectomy for non-small cell lung cancer (NSCLC): Long-term oncologic results. The Journal of Thoracic and Cardiovascular Surgery. 2012;**143**(2):383-389

[39] Cerfolio RJ, Watson C, Minnich DJ, Calloway S, Wei B. One hundred planned robotic segmentectomies: Early results, technical details, and preferred Port placement. The Annals of Thoracic Surgery. 2016 Mar;**101**(3):1089-1095; Discussion 1095-1096. DOI: 10.1016/j.

athoracsur.2015.08.092. [Epub: 02 February 2016]

[40] Kao MC, Lan CH, Huang CJ. Anesthesia for awake video-assisted thoracic surgery. Acta Anaesthesiologica Taiwanica: Official Journal of the Taiwan Society of Anesthesiologists. 2012;**50**(3):126-130

[41] Pompeo E, Tacconi F, Mineo D, Mineo TC. The role of awake video-assisted thoracoscopic surgery in spontaneous pneumothorax. The Journal of Thoracic and Cardiovascular Surgery. 2007;**133**(3):786-790

[42] Tacconi F, Pompeo E, Fabbi E, Mineo TC. Awake video-assisted pleural decortication for empyema thoracis. European Journal of Cardio-Thoracic Surgery: Official Journal of the European Association for Cardio-Thoracic Surgery. 2010;**37**(3):594-601

[43] Chen KC, Cheng YJ, Hung MH, Tseng YD, Chen JS. Nonintubated thoracoscopic lung resection: A 3-year experience with 285 cases in a single institution. Journal of Thoracic Disease. 2012;**4**(4):347-351

[44] Chen JS, Cheng YJ, Hung MH, Tseng YD, Chen KC, Lee YC. Nonintubated thoracoscopic lobectomy for lung cancer. Annals of Surgery. 2011;**254**(6):1038-1043

Chapter 10

Surgical Management of Bronchiectasis

Yasser Ali Kamal

Abstract

Bronchiectasis is a chronic clinicopathological disease of the lung characterized by chronic cough, sputum production, recurrent pulmonary infection, and persistent bronchial dilatation on computed tomography. For many years, bronchiectasis associated with high mortality and morbidity particularly before the advent of antibiotics. The medical treatment of bronchiectasis includes antibiotic therapy, airway clearance, bronchodilators, and anti-inflammatory agents. Surgery is mainly performed for localized disease after failure of the medical treatment, including: segmentectomy, lobectomy, and pneumonectomy. This chapter highlights the current surgical considerations for treatment of bronchiectasis, regarding indications of surgery, preoperative evaluation and preparation, available operative procedures, postoperative outcomes, and other important surgical issues.

Keywords: lung, bronchiectasis, productive cough, thoracic surgery, lung resection

1. Introduction

Bronchiectasis was originally described by René Laënnec in 1819. This term comes from two Greek words; "Bronkhia" and "Ektasis" meaning "Airway widening". As a medical term, bronchiectasis refers to chronic lung disease associated with irreversible dilatation of the bronchial tree. For many years, it was considered as an orphan disease; however, the detection of bronchiectasis has been increased in the recent years as a result of increased health awareness and modern advances in the imaging techniques [1, 2].

The prevalence of bronchiectasis varies in relation to geographic location. The estimated prevalence of bronchiectasis in developed countries (USA, UK, Germany, Spain) is up to 566 cases per 100,000, with 40% increase in the past decade [3, 4]. The recent findings from the British lung foundation's project showed that around 212,000 people are currently living with bronchiectasis in the UK, with predominence of female gender and over-70 age [5]. In USA, 252,362 patients were indentified with an average annual prevalence of 701 per 100,000 persons between 2006 and 2014, with mean age of 76 years, predominace of female gender (65%), and dual diagnosis of chronic obstructive pulmonary disease (COPD) in most of the patients (51%) [6]. In China, the overall prevalence of physician-diagnosed bronchiectasis in people aged 40 years or older is estimated at 1.2% and is trending upward with aging of the population [7]. In comparison to European estimates, the recently reported patients with bronchiectasis in India were younger (median age of 56 years), more likely to be men, and showed a high frequency of severe, cystic bronchiectasis. Tuberculosis and other severe infections were the most frequently reported underlying cause [8].

Most of the cases of bronchiectasis are idiopathic in etiology, however, it may be found in a variety of pulmonary diseases, genetic or acquired, such as cystic fibrosis (CF), Kartagener syndrome (triad of situs inversus, chronic sinusitis, and bronchiectasis), COPD, alpha 1-antitrypsin deficiency, bronchial asthma, or primary immunodeficiencies [9, 10]. In the absence of CF, particularly with post-infectious and allergic hypersensitivity causes, the disease is known as non-cystic fibrosis bronchiectasis (NCFB) [10].

The pathogenesis of bronchiectasis is based on the "vicious cycle hypothesis" which begins by infectious or noninfectious insult to the lung, resulting in neutrophil inflammation (proteases) and impairment of the mucociliary clearance followed by microbial colonization or infection, bronchial obstruction, and exaggerated inflammatory response. The "vicious cycle" (**Figure 1**) refers to the occurrence of repeated infections with repeated impairment of the mucociliary apparatus subsequent to infection and inflammation [10–12].

The clinical diagnosis of bronchiectasis is challenging as it manifests early non-specific symptoms and signs. However, the presence of chronic cough with overproduction of sputum which may worse at the morning increases the index of suspicion for bronchiectasis especially in non-smokers [13, 14]. Other significant signs of bronchiectasis include: hemoptysis, chronic respiratory failure, pulmonary hypertension, and right-sided heart failure [13].

Bronchiectasis can be classified anatomically (cylindrical, varicoid, or cystic), and radiologically (localized or diffuse) [14]. Chest radiographs show non-specific findings of bronchiectasis such as: atelectatic changes, and hyperinflation [13, 14]. High-resolution computed tomography (HRCT) of the chest is a useful imaging tool for diagnosis of bronchiectasis and detection of the underlying causes. On HRCT, bronchiectatic changes include dilated airways, thick-walled bronchi with failed tapering at the periphery of the lung,, ring opacity, tram-track sign, and finger-in-glove sign, and signet-ring sign when the dilated bronchi is larger than the companion pulmonary artery branch (Bronchial-to-arterial ratio > 1) [14].

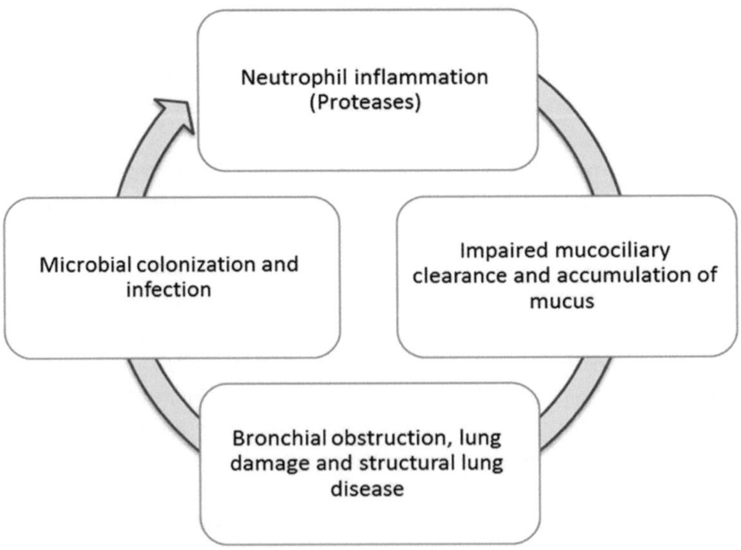

Figure 1.
Vicious cycle of bronchiectasis.

A bundle of minimum etiological tests has been recommended by European Respiratory Society (ERS) for newly diagnosed patients with bronchiectasis including: differential blood count, immunoglobulins (IgA, IgM and IgG), and allergic bronchopulmonary aspergillosis (ABPA)-specific tests (total IgE, specific IgE to Aspergillus, IgG to Aspergillus and eosinophil count), in addition to sputum culture for monitoring of bacterial and non-tuberculous infections [15].

Etiology-specific investigations include: Sweat chloride assessment and cystic fibrosis transmembrane conductance regulator (CFTR) genetic analysis for cystic fibrosis, serum alpha1-antitrypsin level and phenotyping for Alpha-1-antitrypsin deficiency, measurement of nasal nitric oxide levels and ciliated epithelial biopsy for primary ciliary dyskinesia, Rheumatoid factor and anti-cyclic citrullinated peptide (CCP) for autoimmune/connective tissue diseases, and specific CT findings of congenital malformations including Williams-Campbell syndrome (bronchomalacia); Mounier-Kuhn syndrome (tracheobronchomegaly) and lung sequestration [16].

Bronchoscopy is not a routine diagnostic tool for bronchiectasis in the era of HRCT, but there are several indications for diagnostic bronchoscopy in such cases including: exclusion of foreign body obstruction especially in children, exclusion of proximal obstruction in adults with localized disease, obtaining microbiological results in acute ill patients, sampling of lower respiratory tract secretions when serial sputum testing did not yield results, obtaining endobronchial biopsy of airway cilia, and localizing the site of bleeding in patients with bronchiectasis and hemoptysis [17].

The age-adjusted mortality rate for both male and female patients with diagnosed bronchiectasis is more than twice the mortality in the general population [4]. The independent risk factors influencing long-term mortality (over 13 years) in patients with bronchiectasis include: age, St George's Respiratory Questionnaire activity score, *Pseudomonas aeruginosa* infection, total lung capacity (TLC), residual volume/TLC, and the transfer factor coefficient [18]. Therefore, in order to reduce the suspected poor prognosis with bronchiectasis, the treatment should be directed to improve symptoms, enhance quality of life, reduce exacerbations, and limit progression of the bronchiectatic lesions [15, 19].

Treatment of bronchiectasis has been considered by ERS guidelines according to the vicious cycle hypothesis [15]. Thus, the options of treatment include: long-term inhaled or oral antibiotic therapy, eradication of new pathogenic microorganisms and antibiotic treatment of exacerbations for chronic bronchial infection, long-term anti-inflammatory therapies for inflammation, long-term mucoactive treatments and airway clearance techniques for impaired mucociliary clearance, and long-term bronchodilator therapy, surgery and pulmonary rehabilitation for structural lung disease.

2. Indications of surgery

Optimization of the medical management and proper selection of patients are crucial in the decesion making for surgery. Therefore, the current guidelines by ERS and British Thoracic Society (BTS) did not consider surgery until the symptoms are controlled by optimized medical treatment [15, 20]. The indications of surgery as recently mentioned by BTS guideline (**Figure 2**) include: persistent symptoms despite up to a year of comprehensive medical treatment, exacerbations that are either severe or frequent and interfere with social/professional life, recurrent refractory or massive hemoptysis, post obstruction bronchiectasis distal to tumors, localized severely damaged lobe/segment that may be a source of sepsis that left in situ may lead to extension of lung damage, and treatment of complications such as empyema or lung abscess [20].

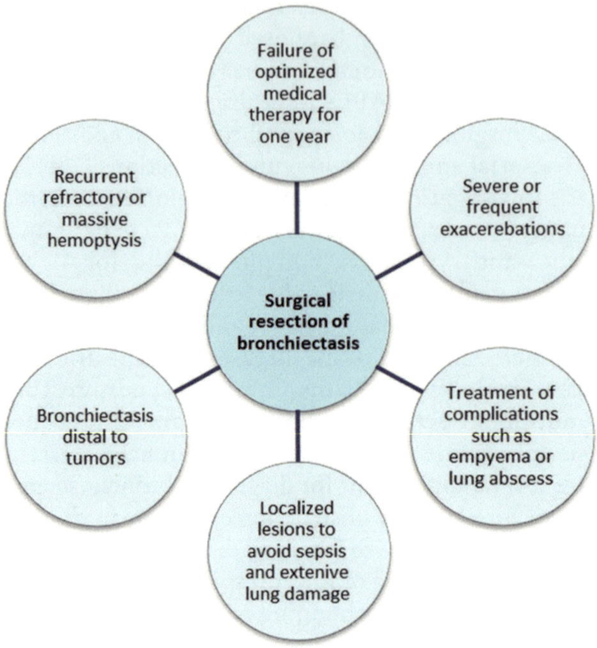

Figure 2.
Current indications for surgical treatment of bronchiectasis [15, 20].

Up to date, there are only 46 published studies in literature between 1960 and 2019, evaluating the surgical management of bronchiectasis [21–66]. The most common clinical manifestations in these studies were: productive cough in 17.4–100% [54, 57], fetid sputum in 15.1–80% [35, 57], and hemoptysis in 10–76.5% [44, 59], while the main and indications of surgery include: failure of medical therapy in 39.6–100% [43, 50], recurrent chest infection in 19.8–100% [23, 54], massive or recurrent hemoptysis in 3–44.3% [32, 43], lung abscess in 1.8–36.5% [32, 58], lung masses or tumors in 1.4–17.6% [42, 46], and empyema in 1.1–8.1% [30, 57]. The mean duration of symptoms before surgery ranged from 1.78–10.6 years [30, 66].

Failure of prudent medical treatment is the main indication of surgery in these studies, especially with frequent exacerbations and repeated hospitalizations [41]. Some authors considered failure of treatment if sputum production persists after 2 or 3 cycles of treatment [35]. The permanently damaged areas of bronchiectasis have poor antibiotic penetration leading to failure of antibiotic therapy, and acts as a microbiological reservoir with subsequent recurrence of infection [61]. Moreover, medical treatment for long periods with persistent symptoms has additional psychological and social effects [32].

Therefore, surgery after failed medical treatment should aim to improve clinical condition and health-related quality of life, in addition to resolution of terrible bronchiectasis-related complications. This aim can be achieved when the focal lesions are completely removed, however, patients with multisegmental lesions should have palliative limited resection after failure of medical treatment or in the presence of life-threatening hemoptysis [47].

Recurrence of pulmonary infection is an important indication of surgery, as it can result in increased cost and side effects of antibiotic therapy for acute infection, in addition to affection of the normal lung tissue with extension of lung destruction during each episode [32]. When bronchiectasis is associated with lung abscess, surgery should be delayed until adequate control with antibiotic therapy and avoiding of preoperative drainage is recommended, however, the immediate indications of surgery in the presence of lung abscess include increased abscess size, unceasing sepsis, and contralateral contamination [30].

Recurrent or massive hemoptysis of more than 600 mL of blood within 24 hours indicates surgery which is considered as emergency after failure of the conservative therapy for hemoptysis. Even after initial cessation of bleeding by balloon blockade of the bleeding bronchus or bronchial artery embolization, early surgical treatment is indicated to avoid life-threatening recurrence of hemoptysis [30].

In children, the indications for surgery are the same as in adult patients. Growth retardation can be considered as an additional indication for surgery in children with satisfactory postoperative results [43]. It is crucial to exclude the underlying diseases such as Kartagener syndrome and cystic fibrosis which limit the surgical resection [36].

3. Preoperative evaluation

Preoperative evaluation should include physical examination, imaging studies, arterial blood gases, pulmonary function tests, bronchoscopy, and perfusion scans if indicated. Additional diagnostic work-up may be required for patients with cardiovascular diseases including echocardiography, stress testing, myocardial perfusion studies, and coronary angiography [48].

3.1 Chest radiography

Chest radiography represents non-specific features of bronchiectasis with low sensitivity and difficult appreciation. The suggestive findings in moderate to severe patients include: stranding, cystic lesions, volume loss with crowding of vessels, atelectasis, tram-track appearance, ring-like opacities, and tubular densities [28, 67]. Despite inadequate role of chest radiography in evaluation of bronchiectasis, abnormalities on chest radiography is significantly correlated with severity of the disease on HRCT [68].

3.2 High resolution computed tomography (HRCT)

The images of HRCT have higher sensitivity for diagnosis and localization of bronchiectasis than radiography with very low false negative and false positive results [41, 69]. The indications of HRCT include: clinical suspicion despite normal chest radiography, clarification of abnormalities on chest radiography, and decision making for surgery [70]. The use of HRCT is not restricted by age of the patient, thus HRCT is not uncommon diagnostic tool in children with bronchiectasis [56].

In addition to the great help of HRCT in diagnosis of different types of bronchiectasis (**Figure 3**), preoperative localization of the lesions by HRCT has specific importance in making the decision for complete anatomic resection or limited resection with preservation of the lung tissue [30].

3.3 Bronchoscopy

Bronchoscopy should be performed in all patients to determine the underlying causes of bronchial obstruction including: foreign body aspiration, endobronchial epithelial tumors, and enlarged hilar lymph nodes with lobar collapse [30, 36].

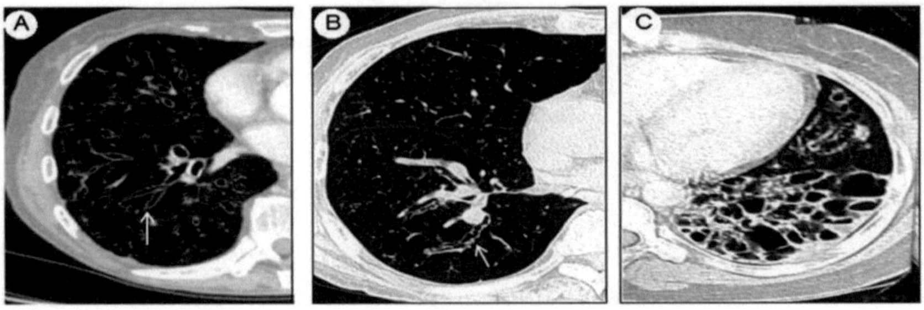

Figure 3.
Images of high resolution computed tomography show types of bronchiectasis: (A) cylindrical, (B) varicose, and (C) cystic.

Preoperative removal of the secretions and clearing of the airways is an important indication of bronchoscopy in adult and children patients [63], as it is associated with lower rate of postoperative complications [41].

3.4 Pulmonary function tests

Pulmonary function tests (PFTs) are not routinely performed in cases of bronchiectasis when the lesions are localized, but PFTs should be performed in diffuse bronchiectasis and in cases of repeated operations [36]. Pulmonary function tests can be performed in adult patients or in children older than 6 years of age [59]; however, cooperation of the child may affect completeness of the pulmonary function tests [35].

The patients with bronchiectasis may have obstructive ventilatory pattern related to mucus retention or immunological abnormalities. The surgical resection of pulmonary segments with little contribution to ventilatory process is expected to have no or minimal effect on postoperative pulmonary function [31]. The expected loss of pulmonary function after surgical resection of bronchiectasis can be calculated from the equation: expected loss of function = preoperative function * (number of functional segments in the lobe to be resected/total number of segments of both lungs) [53].

3.5 Perfusion scans (ventilation/perfusion scintigraphy)

Ventilation/perfusion (V/Q) scintigraphy provides information about hemodynamic features (vascular perfusion), gas exchange, and quantitative lung function, which has a particular help in cases with diffuse bronchiectasis as it can determine the most affected non-perfused areas to be surgically resected [36, 37]. The affected area is considered non-perfused when the perfusion is <10% of the expected [37]. Moreover, V/Q scintigraphy is indicated in patients with poor pulmonary function to provide more quantitative information about ventilation function [38].

Some authors tried to find the correlation between morphologic type of bronchiectasis and the hemodynamic perfusion features. The study by Ashour in 1996, determined a correlation of cylindric morphology with pulmonary perfusion, contrary to non-perfusion predominance in cystic type, thus the surgery for diffuse bronchiectasis can be reserved for non-perfused cystic lesions which are more damaged than cylindrical lesions [71]. Thereafter, Al-Kattan and colleagues reported a new hemodynamic classification of bronchiectasis in patients with diffuse or bilateral disease, combining the perfusion and morphologic features to provide a reasonable extent of surgery and to obtain maximum postoperative clinical improvement [37].

4. Preoperative preparation

The preoperative preparation of patients with bronchiectasis should aim to provide the best possible status. Therefore, the preoperative preparation should be performed by a multidisciplinary team consists of infectious disease specialists, pulmonologists, and thoracic surgeons [72].

4.1 Sputum culture analysis

The patients should have appropriate preoperative preparation until the sputum volume reduced to 20-50 mL per day [54, 63], or the antibiotic therapy is modified according to new culture sensitivity results of the sputum [63]. As the gram-negative bacterial infection has a significant risk for perioperative complications, surgery should be performed after negative proof of Gram-negative bacillus on sputum culture analysis [58].

In patients with a history of tuberculosis, surgery should be reserved for patients with inactive disease. Some surgeons postponed elective surgery 6 months if the sputum culture was positive for acid-fast bacilli and after the completion of antituberculosis treatment [41].

4.2 Infection control

Preoperatively, patients should be hospitalized and prepared for at least 2 weeks before surgery [48]. The patients who are scheduled for surgery should have no active pulmonary infection at the time of surgery. Therefore, broadspectrum antibiotics should be given for 48 hours prior to surgery, or prophylactic antibiotics are given according to results of sputum culture and sensitivity tests [36, 54]. For prophylaxis, cephalosporin and aminoglycoside are preferred if the culture is negative and the patient has no contraindications or allergies [48].

4.3 Chest physiotherapy and postural drainage

The patients should have intensive chest physiotherapy in the preoperative period, to obtain acceptable decrease of the daily volume of the sputum [54]. Patients should have chest physiotherapy including postural drainage for at least 2 weeks bfore surgery [57], or it should be continued until the daily sputum is ≤50 mL [50]. Preoperative postural drainage is essential to clean intra-tracheal secretions, decrease the sputum volume and sputum accumulation, and hence control of the infection and optimize the respiratory status [50, 58].

The recommended airway clearance techniques are active breathing techniques or oscillating positive expiratory pressure (PEP). Review of HRCT findings is helpful to determine the appropriate postural drainage in relevance to the affected pulmonary segments. The gravity assisted positioning, where not contraindicated, is recommended to enhance the effectiveness of an airway clearance technique. Modified postural drainage without head down tilt should be considered when the postural drainage is not tolerated and when the symptoms of gastroesophageal reflux increased with the technique [17, 20].

4.4 Other considerations

Nutritional support and pulmonary rehabilitation should be considered before surgical referral [20]. In patients on long-term steroid therapy, the doses may be increased by 5–10 mg/day, but surgery should be postponed in patients with uncontrolled respiratory symptoms [72].

5. Surgical procedures

5.1 Thoracotomy

The anesthetic management during surgery for bronchiectasis should consider: (1) cleaning of the bronchus opposite to the side of surgery by aspiration before placement of endotracheal tube, and (2) avoiding contralateral contamination by: insertion of double-lumen endotracheal tube, use of Fogarty embolectomy catheter as a bronchus blocker, or advancing of the endotracheal tube to the main bronchus of the opposite side of resection [35, 37, 41, 54, 57].

Posterolateral thoracotomy is the standard approach for pulmonary resection in patients with bronchiectasis. Preservation of the integrity of chest wall muscles using muscle-sparing technique is essential to reduce postoperative pain and generate an effective cough [29]. When the decision is for bilateral lung resection, the second operation can be performed with an interval of 1–4 months [49, 53].

The extent of lung resection is determined by extent of the disease and cardiopulmonary reserve, thus lobectomy is performed for lesions limited to one lobe, segmentectomy is performed for fairly limited disease or when the pulmonary function is impaired, while pneumonectomy is reserved for extensive disease affecting the whole lung [33, 50, 54]. In some instances, bilobectomy and lobectomy plus segmentectomy can be performed [40, 44, 48, 50, 52, 61]. Extrapleural dissection is preferred to avoid spillage of lung content into pleural space. After identification of the hilar structures and opening of the major fissure, arterial, venous, and bronchial branches are isolated and divided, respectively [39, 63].

Certain recommendations can be followed to prevent or reduce the incidences of postoperative air leak and bronchopleural fistula (BPF) after lung resection including: preservation of peribronchial tissues and avoidance of extensive lymph node dissection near to bronchi to minimize bronchial devascularization, division of the bronchus before mobilization of the resected part to avoid contamination of the healthy segments, division of the bronchial stump as short as possible which sutured by non-absorbable materials or closed with a mechanical stapler then buttressed by tissue glue or a flap from pleura, pericardium, pericardial fat pad, muscle, or omentum [41, 73].

To reduce the extension of contamination during surgery, extrapleural intrapericardial pneumonectomy is recommended when there is pleural sepsis or complete fusion of the pleura. Also, the evidence of pleural infection indicates pleural space irrigation with antibiotic [73]. Following placement of the chest drains, bronchoscopic evaluation of the bronchial sutures with removal of any secretions in the airway should be performed [63]. The resected specimens should be sent for histopathological examination [41].

5.2 Video-assisted thoracoscopic surgery (VATS)

There is a little research work regarding use of VATS in the management of bronchiectasis. The reported VATS approaches for lobectomy in patients with bronchiectasis include three ports, two ports, or one port VATS [55, 62, 66]. Additionally, a two-port thoracoscopy with a utility mini-thoracotomy has been reported [45].

For three ports completely VATS procedure, the ports are placed through the 7th or 8th intercostal space in the midaxillary line for a 10-mm 30° thoracoscope, the 4th or 5th intercostal space along the anterior axillary line (4–5 cm incision), and the 7th or 8th intercostal space in the auscultatory triangle (1.5 cm incision) [55]. For two ports VATS lobectomy, a 2 cm camera port through the 7th or 8th intercostal space in the anterior axillary line and a 3–5 cm utility incision through the 4th or 5th intercostal space in the anterior or mid axillary line [62]. Ocakcioglu et al. described uniportal VATS lobectomy through a utility incision of 3–5 cm from the 5th intercostal space in the anterior position without use of rib retractor. A 10 mm 30° thoracoscope is placed in the anterior part of the incision, while dissecting and holding clamps are placed through the dorsal part [66].

During 3 ports VATS, the incisions change depending on the type of lung resection, whether it is an upper or lower lobectomy [62]. The presence of intrathoracic adhesions is a challenging problem during VATS which can be released by blunt or sharp dissection, or it may result in conversion of the VATS procedure to open procedure [55, 64]. As in open thoracotomy, the pulmonary artery is firstly identified and divided before the division of the veins to avoid congestion of the lobe, with separate dissection of the major pulmonary veins and the bronchus [64]. The dissection of vascular and airway structures is performed by an endoscopic linear cutter [55]. At the end of VATS procedure, the thorax is closed after retrieval of the resected specimens and meticulous control of air leak and hemorrhage [66].

5.3 Postoperative care

Bronchoscopy can be performed in the operating room for bronchial hygiene, immediately after surgery [56]. The early postoperative care should include: pain control including epidural analgesia, chest physiotherapy, antibiotic therapy according to results of culture and sensitivity [37, 56].

Generally, the duration of postoperative systematic antibiotic therapy is 5 days, but it can be longer according to the inflammatory condition. Early ambulation and active cough, and 3–4 times percussive chest physiotherapy are essential for proper expectoration and lung re-expansion. The standard criteria for removal of chest tube are: stable vital signs, small amount of drainage (<100 mL/day) with clear color, lung re-expansion on chest X-ray, and absence of air leak [63].

After discharge, patients should have specific or wide-spectrum antibiotic therapy for 1 week. Chest physiotherapy can be reinitiated at home and continued for 2 weeks after discharge [33].

6. Postoperative outcomes of lung resection

6.1 Mortality

To date, few studies have evaluated postoperative outcomes after lung resection for bronchiectasis (**Table 1**). There is no perioperative mortality (early, operative, in-hospital, postoperative, or 30-days) after surgical resection of bronchiectasis in most of the published studies. The reported rates of perioperative mortality ranged from 0.41% [23] to 8.3% [25]. The causes of early mortality in literature include: respiratory failure [2, 27, 28, 41, 49, 57], intraoperative bleeding [24, 28, 46], postoperative pneumonia [25, 37], empyema [25, 32], pulmonary edema [27, 46], cardiac-related causes including myocardial infarction or arrhythmia [27, 35, 47, 49, 58], speptic shock [27, 56], gastrointestinal bleeding due to sepsis and stress ulcer [39], uncontrolled hemoptysis [27], pulmonary embolism [22, 32, 48, 58], cardiac arrest in patients with Kartagener syndrome [36], disseminated intravascular coagulation [44], nephropathy [22], downstream consequences of bronchial stump fistula [48, 60], multiple organ failure [48, 60], and causes unrelated to disease or technique such as cerebral edema in a child due to previously undiagnosed aquaeductus stenosis and hydrocephalus [24]. The disease-related consequences which indirectly attribute to early death include: severe disease requiring

Author	Year	Number	Morbidity (%)	Early mortality (%)	Late mortality (%)	Asymptomatic (%)
Hewlett and Ziperman	1960	107	20.6	0	1.9	36.4
Streete and Salyer	1960	240	22.1	0.8	2.1	22.3
Sanderson et al.	1974	242	33.5	0.4	2.9	62.5
George et al.	1979	99	88.9	3	4	39.6
Annest et al.	1982	24	12.5	8.3	8.3	45.8
Wilson and Decker	1982	84	10.7	0	1.2	73.8
Dogan et al.	1989	487	10.7	3.1	0.4	73.3
Agasthian et al.	1996	134	24.6	2.2	0	59.2
Ashour et al.	1999	85	12.9	0	0	74.1
Fujimoto et al.	2001	90	22.2	0	0	45.6
Prieto et al.	2001	119	12.6	0	0	67.6
Kutlay et al.	2002	166	10.8	1.8	0	75
Balkanli et al.	2003	238	8.8	0	0	82.5
Mazieres et al.	2003	16	18.8	0	0	31.3
Haciibrahimoglu et a	2004	35	17.1	2.9	0	64.7
Otgun et al.	2004	54	7.4	5.6	0	45.1
Al-Kattan et al.	2005	66	18.2	1.5	0	73.8
Schneiter et al.	2005	48	18.8	0	0	62.5
Aghajanzadeh et al.	2006	29	37.9	3.4	0	67.9
Yuncu et al.	2006	81	18.5	0	0	81.7
Eren et al.	2007	143	23.1	1.4	0	75.9
Guerra et al.	2007	51	15.7	0	0	77.8
Sirmali et al	2007	176	13.1	0	0	73.3
Stephen et al.	2007	149	14.8	0.7	0.7	54.3
Giovannetti et al.	2008	45	11.1	0	0	71.1
Bagheri et al.	2010	277	15.9	0.7	0	68.6
Gursoy et al.	2010	92	16.3	1.1	0	84
Zhang et al.	2010	790	16.2	1.1	0	67.7
Caylak et al.	2011	339	12.7	0.6	0	71
Cobanoglu et al.	2011	62	19.4	0	0	45
Gorur et al.	2011	122	13.1	0	0	77.3
Sehitogullari et al.	2011	129	22.5	0	0.8	60.2
Hiramatsu et al.	2012	31	19.4	0	0	74.2
Al-Refaie et al.	2013	138	13	0	0	84.2
Zhou et al.	2013	56	23.2	0	0	58.9

Author	Year	Number	Morbidity (%)	Early mortality (%)	Late mortality (%)	Asymptomatic (%)
Andrade et al.	2014	109	36.7	0.9	0.9	NR
Balci et al.	2014	86	16.3	1.2	0	82.6
Jin et al.	2014	260	11.5	0.8	1.9	78
Sahin et al.	2014	60	20	0	3.3	74.1
Vallilo et al.	2014	53	24.5	3.8	0	34.1
Coutinho et al.	2016	69	14.5	0	0	73.3
Baysungur et al.	2017	41	9.8	0	0	NR
Dai et al.	2017	37	21.6	0	0	62.2
Hao et al.	2019	99	17.2	0	0	26
Nega et al.	2019	22	22.7	4.5	0	89.5
Ocakcioglu et al.	2019	14	14.3	0	0	85.7

NR: Not reported.

Table 1.
Reported outcomes (%) after surgical treatment of bronchiectasis [21–66].

pneumonectomy or completion [28, 58], massive bleeding during the operation because of dense adhesions due to chronic and recurrent infections [44, 46], and Kartagener syndrome [36].

The rates of late or long-term mortality ranged from 0.41% [27] to 8.3% [25]. The reported causes of late mortality after surgical management of bronchiectasis included: respiratory failure [24, 52], progressive respiratory disease [25], sepsis [59], coronary artery thrombosis [22], cor pulmonale or pulmonary heart disease [22, 58], myocardial failure [22], glomerulonephritis [22], kidney failure [58], post-pneumonectomy pneumonia in the remaining lung [56], massive bleeding from the Malecot catheter used for drainage ofresidual space infection [44], suicide [22], and other causes of late deaths not attributable to bronchiectasis [21, 23, 26].

6.2 Morbidity

The reported rates of morbidity ranged from 7% [7] to 38% [39]. The most common complication is atelectasis or sputum retention requiring bronchoscopic intervention, followed by persistent air leak (**Table 2**). Most of the reported complications were minor, transient, and treatable.

In comparison to the published studies in the 3rd and 4th decades of 20th century, the relatively low incidences of complication in the after while studies can reflect effective antibiotic therapy, improved anesthetic techniques, adequate blood transfusion, and detailed postoperative care [21, 22]. Other factors include: surgeon's experience, preoperative awareness of the undesirable consequences of retained secretions, preoperative teaching of breathing exercises, scheduling tracheal suction or bronchoscopy in the early postoperative period [21], good intra-operative hemostasis and careful dissection [37], low number of pneumonectomies, accurate patient selection, and careful perioperative management [45].

Treatment of postoperative complications after surgery for bronchiectasis depends on its type and severity. The treatment options for complications include: physiotherapy, tube thoracotomy, bronchoscopic treatment for atelectasis, negative suction applied to the chest tubes for prolonged air leak, surgical reintervention for closure

Complications	Minimum rate [Reference]	Maximum rate [Reference]
Atelectasis or sputum retention	0.9% [21]	33.3% [24]
Prolonged air leak	0.7% [54]	26.4% [23]
Pneumonia	1.2% [57]	12.5% [34]
Bronchopleural fistula	0.4% [48]	9.1% [65]
Residual air space or expansion defect	2.2% [45]	9% [51]
Empyema	0.6% [32]	8.1% [44]
Wound infection	1.3% [44]	7.4% [27]
Bleeding	1.1% [30]	8.3% [25]
Cardiac arrhythmias	0.4% [58]	5.4% [63]
Pulmonary embolism	0.4% [58]	3.8% [60]
Respiratory insufficiency	0.8% [52]	3.5% [57]
Pulmonary edema	0.8% [52]	2.2% [28]
Pleural effusion	0.6% [32]	0.7% [54]

Table 2.
Reported rates of complications after surgical treatment of bronchiectasis.

of bronchopleural fistula, medical treatment or decortication for pleural empyema, pharmacological control of supraventricular arrhythmias, reexploration for postoperative bleeding, and mechanical ventilation for respiratory insufficiency [39, 41, 60].

Cobanoglu et al. did not report any significant statistical difference between tubular and saccular morphologic types of bronchiectasis regarding postoperative complication rates; however, the most severe postoperative complication, bronchopleural fistula, developed in 2 (3.22%) cases with saccular bronchiectasis [50]. Zhou et al. did not find statistically significant difference in the rates of postoperative complications between thoracotomy and VATS procedure. Minor postoperative complications were reported after thoracotomy or completely VATS lobectomy, which included pneumonia, prolonged air leak (>7 days), and atelectasis [55]. Moreover, Hao et al. did not observe major postoperative complications such as bronchopleural fistula or respiratory insufficiency was observed in VATS and thoracotomy groups. The most common complication was persistent air leak for >7 days in 8.1% of VATS group and 6% of thoracotomy group [64].

6.3 Symptomatic improvement

The clinical results after surgical resection of bronchiectasis are frequently classified into three categories. The first category (asymptomatic; excellent response) includes patients who are completely free of any symptoms suggestive of bronchiectasis, and considered themselves cured. The second category (clinical improvement; good response) includes those considered improved who have had some relief of the symptoms but still had some chronic pulmonary complaints. The third category (no improvement; poor response) includes patients with no-change, no-reduction in preoperative symptoms, or who are worse off since surgical resection. [22, 31, 32, 35, 44, 46, 47, 50]. Some authors referred to the excellent response as well outcome [36] or perfect response [41].

Sanderson et al. expanded the classification of the clinical symptomatic outcome to five categories as: excellent (no symptoms at all), good (full physical capacity, occasional cough and sputum), fair-improved (tendency to cough and sputum with susceptibility to respiratory infection, hemoptysis or dyspnea), poor (residual symptoms), and worse (steady deterioration) [23]. Other authors reduced the classification of the clinical condition in two categories only by dividing the patients into an improved group ("excellent" or "good" outcomes) and an unimproved group ("no change" or "worse" outcomes) [52].

In literature, through a range of follow-up between 9 months and 14 years, the proportion of asymptomatic patients or excellent improvement after surgery ranged from 22.3% [22] to 89.5% [65], while the proportion of clinical improvement with reduction of preoperative symptoms ranged from 9.6% [64] to 80.7% [56], and no improvement, worseness or relapse was reported in 1.6% [58] to 42.3% [22].

6.4 Quality of life (QOL)

Patients with bronchiectasis report worse quality of life (QOL) than do persons in the general population [74, 75]. Recurrent bronchiectasis exacerbations are related to deterioration of lung function, progression of the disease, impairment of quality of life, and increased rate of mortality [76]. Postoperative QOL and the functional consequences of lung resection (pulmonary function and exercise capacity) are poorly addressed.

Vallilo et al. reported a significant improvement of the QOL in patients with symptomatic bronchiectasis which was particularly relevant in the functional and physical QOL domains. Resection of the lung area which had not contributed to ventilatory response during exercise before surgery might enable the patients to maintain the exercise performance after lung resection without impairment to the response of the ventilatory system during maximal testing [60].

6.5 Complete versus incomplete resection

The proper surgical treatment should aim to complete resection of the bronchiectatic lesions. Thus, intraoperatively detected lesions should be resected as appropriate whether determined on preoperative imaging studies or not [32]. Complete resection is defined as an anatomic resection of all affected segments preoperatively identified by high-resolution computed tomography or bronchography [48, 54, 57]. However, some authors considered pulmonary resection complete if the patient was believed to be free of bronchiectasis after thoracotomy [31, 35].

Completeness of surgical resection is affected by localization of the disease and pulmonary function (**Figure 4**). In patients with unilateral localized bronchiectasis, the most important prognostic factor for good surgical outcomes is complete resection of all diseased segments. In bilateral localized bronchiectasis, complete surgical resection should be attempted if lung function permits, including combinations of lobectomy with segmentectomy or wedge resections on the same siting or staged [24, 39, 73]; however, limited resection of the most predominant lesion is preferred for selected patients with bilateral diffuse bronchiectasis [34, 63]. The reported completeness of resection in patients with localized bronchiectasis ranged from 55.4% [23] to 94.2% [54].

Sanderson et al. found a preponderance of excellent results after complete resection in comparison with incomplete resection (36% versus 10%, $P < 0.005$) [23]. Agasthian et al. found that complete resection resulted in a significant increase in proportion of asymptomatic patients than incomplete resection (65.2% versus 21.4%, $p < 0.05$) [28]. In the study by Kutlay et al., the excellent to good results of complete resection were significantly better than those of incomplete resection (98.5 versus 76.5%, $P < 0.05$) [32]. Similarly, other authors reported significantly better clinical results with complete resection than incomplete resection [35, 36, 44, 46, 50, 52].

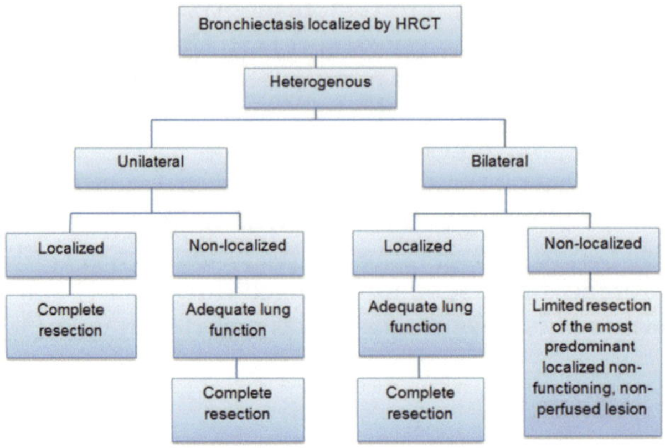

Figure 4.
Simplified algorithm for complete surgical resection according to extent of bronchiectasis.

6.6 Predictors of postoperative outcomes

There is no single independent perioperative variable that can predict occurrence of adverse events after lung resection with scant available data. In the study by Fujimoto et al., the logistic analyses extracted the type of bronchiectasis (cylindrical or others), the history of sinusitis, and the type of resection (complete or incomplete) for discrimination between patients with excellent or improved clinical outcome and patients with no clinical change [30]. Hiramatsu et al. reported immuno compromised status, *Pseudomonas aeruginosa* infection, and extent of residual bronchiectasis, as independent and significant factors of postoperative shorter relapse-free interval [53].

Eren et al. fond that the lack of preoperative bronchoscopic examination, a FEV1 of <60% of the predicted value, a history of tuberculosis, and incomplete resection were independent predictors of postoperative complications [41]. Bagheri et al. statistically evaluated several variables including: sex, age, localization of disease, and complete or incomplete resection using multivariate logistic regression. Complete resection was found to have a significantly better surgical outcome compared to incomplete resection [46]. In the study by Zhang et al., the logistic regression analysis showed that tuberculous bronchiectasis, type of bronchiectasis (saccular versus others), and type of resection (incomplete or complete) were three independent factors associated with poor surgical outcome [48]. The multivariable analyses by Jin et al., showed that age, sputum volume, gram-negative bacillus infection, and bronchial stump coverage were the four independent factors related with poor surgical outcome [58].

According to the reported results by Sahin et al., the prognostic variables in pediatric patients were: FEV1 less than 60% of the predicted value, hemoptysis, and duration of symptoms [59]. Interestingly, Gorur et al. stated that multi-segmental resectable bronchiectasis should not be considered an occult risk factor for morbidity after lung resection. Moreover, the number of resected segments, hemoptysis, and absence of preoperative fiberoptic bronchoscopy were not associated with postoperative complications. Impaired pulmonary function was significantly associated with residual air space; however it did not predict the risk of persistent air leak, atelectasis or empyema [51].

Completion pneumonectomy is historically recognized as a high-risk procedure especially when done for a benign disease [77]. To reduce the high-risk of completion pneumonectomy when indicated, precautions such as optimal exposure, intrapericardial isolation of blood vessels, and bronchial reinforcement are recommended [78]. In the study by Agasthian et al., all died patients after lung resection had completion pneumonectomy. The causes of death were respiratory failure and intraoperative bleeding [28]. However, Fujimoto et al. reported acceptable mortality and morbidity after completion pneumonectomy without mortality and only one patient had postoperative bronchopleural fistula that could be managed conservatively [30].

7. Specific surgical considerations

7.1 Non-localized bronchiectasis

Patients with non-localized (multi-segmental or bilateral) bronchiectasis are generally regarded as an exclusion of surgery [39]. However, considering the limited and palliative effect of medical treatment and the risk of transplantation or radical operation, recent studies offered a limited operation to some of these patients [34, 63]. Moreover, some surgeons favored surgery in non-localized bronchiectasis to prevent extension of the disease to the unaffected lung [38].

George et al. suggested that bilateral bronchiectasis need not be a contraindication to operation. In properly selected patients, lasting symptomatic improvement can be provided by resection [24]. Mazieres et al. reported favorable outcome after a limited lung resection in properly selected symptomatic patients with severe multisegmental bilateral bronchiectasis, particularly those with cystic lesions and functionless territories [34].

Schneiter et al. found the same patients' satisfaction at 6 months after surgery for patients who had resectable non-localized or localized bronchiectasis, with non-significant differences in the rates of recurrent infection and hemoptysis [38]. Aghajanzadeh et al. reported the benefits of surgery in 87 bilateral non-localized bronchiectases, and concluded that staged bilateral resection for bronchiectases can be performed at any age with acceptable morbidity and mortality [39]. Additionally, Dai et al. reported the safety of lobectomy for the predominant lesions in non-localized bronchiectasis, with significant relief of symptoms, good rates of satisfaction, no operative mortality, and minimal postoperative complications [63].

7.2 Surgery for bronchiectasis in children

The prevalence of bronchiectasis in children ranges from 0.2 to 735 cases per 100,000 [79]. Cystic fibrosis is the most common cause of bronchiectasis in developed countries while in developing countries non-CF etiologies particularly post-infectious causes are more common [80]. Surgical treatment of bronchiectasis in children is considered for cases with resectable disease after failure of the proper medical treatment. Moreover, surgery can be considered in children with diffuse disease who have expected benefit after excision of the most predominant lesions [36, 79].

In literature, the studies that evaluate surgical treatment of bronchiectasis in children are scanty. However, these studies confirmed the safety of surgery for childhood bronchiectasis with low rates of mortality and morbidity. Complete resection can be considered when possible, as most of the children can benefit from surgery especially if the total excision is accomplished [26, 35, 36, 43, 56, 59].

The reported surgical outcomes in children with bronchiectasis highlight: acceptable mortality and morbidity [35, 36, 43, 56, 59], significant impact of surgery on improvement of symptoms and quality of life [43, 56], good results after segmentectomy when the pulmonary segment is entirely free of disease [26], increase the chance of cure after complete resection which results in significantly better outcome than incomplete resection [35, 43], preference of pneumonectomy instead of leaving residual disease when bronchiectasis is unilateral [36], and significant impact of duration of symptoms and timely intervention on the management and prognosis [59].

8. Conclusions

Bronchiectasis is a significant chronic lung disease associated with vicious cycle of inflammation, infection, mucus accumulation, and structural tissue damage. Current guidelines recommend surgical treatment of bronchiectasis in patients with localized disease when symptoms are not controlled by optimized medical treatment. Other indications in literature include recurrent refractory or massive hemoptysis, bronchiectasis distal to tumors, and treatment of subsequent complications.

HRCT is the gold standard imaging tool of bronchiectasis, as has a great help in preoperative localization of the lesions which affects the decision making for surgery. Preoperative bronchoscopy is important to diagnose the underlying causes of bronchial obstruction and to clear the airways by removal of secretions. Preoperative PFTs can be performed to determine the segments with little ventilatory contribution and minimal effects on postoperative pulmonary function after surgical resection. Perfusion scans can be used to determine the most affected non-perfused areas to be resected, particularly when the pulmonary function is affected. According to hemodynamic analysis of perfusion scans in diffuse bronchiectasis, surgery can be reserved for non-perfused cystic lesions which are more damaged than cylindrical lesions.

Preoperative preparation for lung resection should include sputum culture analysis to modify antibiotic therapy with culture sensitivity results. It is crucial to eradicate active pulmonary infection and provide prophylactic antibiotic therapy with cephalosporin and aminoglycoside before surgery. Preoperative airway clearance techniques including active breathing, oscillating PEP, and postural drainage, are recommended to control infection and optimize the respiratory status. Other important preoperative considerations include nutritional support and pulmonary rehabilitation.

Posterolateral thoracotomy is the standard approach for the surgical resection of bronchiectasis. The extent of resection depends on extent of the disease and cardiopulmonary reserve. Preservation of peribronchial tissues, short bronchial stump, and buttressing techniques are recommended to reduce postoperative air leak and BPF. The safety and feasibility of VATS in the treatment of bronchiectasis was shown in scant studies with low morbidity and mortality. The proper care after surgery should include bronchoscopic removal of secretions, pain control, chest physiotherapy, and appropriate antibiotic therapy.

In literature, the mortality rates after lung resection range from 0.41% to 8.3%. The most common causes of early mortality are respiratory failure, intraoperative bleeding, postoperative pneumonia, empyema, pulmonary edema, and cardiac-related causes; while the most common causes of late mortality are respiratory failure, progressive respiratory disease, sepsis, coronary artery thrombosis, and cor pulmonale. The morbidity rates range from 7–38%. Atelctasis or sputum retention is the most common postoperative complication, followed by persistent air leak, pneumonia, and BPF. Most of the reported complications are minor, transient, and treatable. During follow-up periods between 9 months and 14 years, the proportion of asymptomatic patients (excellent improvement) after surgery ranges from 22.3% to 89.5%. Postoperative QOL is poorly addressed, but it can be improved after resection of functionless pulmonary segments.

Complete resection of the affected parenchyma results in better clinical outcome than incomplete resection; however, completeness of resection is affected by localization of the disease and pulmonary function. A large number of predictors of surgical outcomes were investigated in literature, including: type of resection, type of bronchiectasis, immuno compromised status, *Pseudomonas aeruginosa* infection, extent of residual bronchiectasis, lack of preoperative bronchoscopic examination, FEV1 < 60% of the predicted value, tuberculosis, hemoptysis, duration of symptoms, age, sputum volume, gram-negative bacillus infection, bronchial stump coverage, and impaired pulmonary function.

Recent studies reported acceptable outcomes after a limited lung resection for the most predominant lesion in properly selected patients with non-localized bronchiectasis. Surgery can be safely performed in children with bronchiectasis, particularly when the disease is resectable disease after failure of the proper medical treatment. Acceptable postoperative rates of mortality and morbidity and a significant symptomatic improvement were reported in children.

Abbreviations

ABPA	allergic bronchopulmonary aspergillosis
BPF	bronchopleural fistula
BTS	British Thoracic Society
CCP	cyclic citrullinated peptide
CF	cystic fibrosis
CFTR	cystic fibrosis transmembrane conductance regulator
COPD	chronic obstructive pulmonary disease
ERS	European Respiratory Society
FEV1	forced expiratory volume in 1 second
HRCT	high resolution computed tomography
NCFB	non-cystic fibrosis bronchiectasis
PEP	positive expiratory pressure
PFTs	pulmonary function tests
QOL	quality of life
TLC	total lung capacity
VATS	video-assisted thoracoscopic surgery

Author details

Yasser Ali Kamal
Department of Cardiothoracic Surgery, Faculty of Medicine, Minia University, El-Minya, Egypt

*Address all correspondence to: yaser_ali_kamal@yahoo.com

References

[1] Goeminne C, De Soyza A. Bronchiectasis: How to be an orphan with many parents. The European Respiratory Journal. 2016;**47**:10-13

[2] Aliberti S, Chalmers JD. Get together to increase awareness in bronchiectasis: A report of the 2nd world bronchiectasis conference. Multidisciplinary Respiratory Medicine. 2018;**13**(Suppl 1):28. DOI: 10.1186/s40248-018-0138-3

[3] Contarini M, Shoemark A, Rademacher J, Finch S, Gramegna A, Gaffuri M, et al. Why, when and how to investigate primary ciliary dyskinesia in adult patients with bronchiectasis. Multidisciplinary Respiratory Medicine. 2018;**13**(Suppl 1):26

[4] Quint JK, Millett ER, Joshi M, Navaratnam V, Thomas SL, Hurst JR, et al. Changes in the incidence, prevalence and mortality of bronchiectasis in the UK from 2004 to 2013: A population-based cohort study. The European Respiratory Journal. 2016;**47**(1):186-193

[5] Snell N, Gibson J, Jarrold I, Quint JK. Epidemiology of bronchiectasis in the UK: Findings from the British lung foundation's 'Respiratory health of the nation' project. Respiratory Medicine. 2019;**158**:21-23

[6] Henkle E, Chan B, Curtis JR, Aksamit TR, Daley CL, Winthrop KL. Characteristics and health-care utilization history of patients with bronchiectasis in US Medicare enrollees with prescription drug plans, 2006 to 2014. Chest. 2018;**154**(6):1311-1320

[7] Lin JL, Xu JF, Qu JM. Bronchiectasis in China. Annals of the American Thoracic Society. 2016;**13**:609-616

[8] Dhar R, Singh S, Talwar D, Mohan M, Tripathi SK, Swarnakar R, et al. Bronchiectasis in India: Results from the European multicentre bronchiectasis audit and research collaboration (EMBARC) and respiratory research network of India registry. The Lancet Global Health. 2019;**7**(9):e1269-e1279

[9] Maselli DJ, Amalakuhan B, Keyt H, Diaz AA. Suspecting non-cystic fibrosis bronchiectasis: What the busy primary care clinician needs to know. International Journal of Clinical Practice. 2017;**71**(2):1-10. DOI: 10.1111/ijcp.12924

[10] Schäfer J, Griese M, Chandrasekaran R, Chotirmall SH, Hartl D. Pathogenesis, imaging and clinical characteristics of CF and non-CF bronchiectasis. BMC Pulmonary Medicine. 2018;**18**(1):79

[11] Cole PJ. Inflammation: A two-edged sword – The model of bronchiectasis. European Journal of Respiratory Diseases. Supplement. 1986;**147**:6-15

[12] Moulton BC, Barker AF. Pathogenesis of bronchiectasis. Clinics in Chest Medicine. 2012;**33**:211-217

[13] Santhosham R. Bronchiectasis. In: Parikh Rajesh PB, editor. Tips and Tricks in Thoracic Surgery. London: Springer-Verlag; 2018. pp. 87-99

[14] Chana ED, Wooten WI III, Hsiehh EWY, Johnstond KL, Shafferd M, et al. Diagnostic evaluation of bronchiectasis. Respiratory Medicine. 2019;**X**(1):100006. DOI: 10.1016/j.yrmex.2019.100006

[15] Polverino E, Goeminne PC, McDonnell MJ, Aliberti S, Marshall SE, Loebinger MR, et al. European Respiratory Society guidelines for the management of adult bronchiectasis. The European Respiratory Journal. 2017;**50**:1700629

[16] Smith MP. Diagnosis and management of bronchiectasis. CMAJ. 2017;**189**:E828-E835. DOI: 10.1503/cmaj.160830

[17] Pasteur MC, Bilton D, Hill AT. British thoracic society guideline for non-CF bronchiectasis. Thorax. 2010;**65**(Suppl 1):i1-i58

[18] Loebinger MR, Wells AU, Hansell DM, Chinyanganya N, Devaraj A, Meister M, et al. Mortality in bronchiectasis: A long-term study assessing the factors influencing survival. The European Respiratory Journal. 2009;**34**(4):843-849. DOI: 10.1183/09031936.00003709

[19] Koser U, Hill A. What's new in the management of adult bronchiectasis? F1000Research. 2017;**6**(F1000 Facultyb Rev):527. DOI: 10.12688/f1000research.10613.1

[20] Hill AT, Sullivan AL, Chalmers JD, De Soyza A, Elborn SJ, Floto AR, et al. British thoracic society guideline for bronchiectasis in adults. Thorax. 2019;**74**(Suppl 1):1-69. DOI: 10.1136/thoraxjnl-2018-212463

[21] Hewlett TH, Ziperman HH. Bronchiectasis: Results of pulmonary resection. The Journal of Thoracic and Cardiovascular Surgery. 1960;**40**:71-78

[22] Streete BG, Salyer JM. Bronchiectasis: An analysis of 240 cases treated by pulmonary resection. The Journal of Thoracic and Cardiovascular Surgery. 1960;**40**:383-392

[23] Sanderson JM, Kennedy MCS, Johnson MF, Manley DCE. Bronchiectasis: Results of surgical and conservative management - a review of 393 cases. Thorax. 1974;**29**:407

[24] George SA, Leonardi HK, Overholt RH. Bilateral pulmonary resection for bronchiectasis: A 40-year experience. The Annals of Thoracic Surgery. 1979;**28**:48-53

[25] Annest LS, Kratz JM, Crawford FA. Current results of treatment of bronchiectasis. The Journal of Thoracic and Cardiovascular Surgery. 1982;**83**:546-550

[26] Wilson JF, Decker AM. The surgical management of childhood bronchiectasis: A review of 96 consecutive pulmonary resections in children with nontuberculous bronchiectasis. Annals of Surgery. 1982;**195**(3):354-363

[27] Dogan R, Alp M, Kaya S, Ayrancioğlu K, Taştepe I, Unlü M, et al. Surgical treatment of bronchiectasis: A collective review of 487 cases. The Thoracic and Cardiovascular Surgeon. 1989;**37**(3):183-186

[28] Agasthian T, Deschamps C, Trastek VF, Allen MS, Pairolero PC. Surgical management of bronchiectasis. The Annals of Thoracic Surgery. 1996;**62**:976-980

[29] Ashour M, Al-Kattan K, Rafay MA, Saja KF, Hajjar W, Al-Fraye AR. Current surgical therapy for bronchiectasis. World Journal of Surgery. 1999;**23**(11):1096-1104

[30] Fujimoto T, Hillejan L, Stamatis G. Current strategy for surgical management of bronchiectasis. The Annals of Thoracic Surgery. 2001;**72**:1711-1715

[31] Prieto D, Bernardo J, Matos MJ, Euge Ânio L, Antunes M. Surgery for bronchiectasis. European Journal of Cardio-Thoracic Surgery. 2001;**20**:19-23

[32] Kutlay H, Cangir AK, Enön S, Sahin E, Akal M, Güngör A, et al. Surgical treatment in bronchiectasis: Analysis of 166 patients. European Journal of Cardio-Thoracic Surgery. 2002;**21**:634-637

[33] Balkanli K, Genc O, Dakak M, Gürkök S, Gözübüyük A, Caylak H, et al. Surgical management of bronchiectasis: Analysis and short-term results in 238 patients. European Journal of Cardio-Thoracic Surgery. 2003;**24**:699-702

[34] Mazieres J, Murris M, Didier A, Giron J, Dahan M, Berjaud J, et al. Limited operation for severe multisegmental bilateral bronchiectasis. The Annals of Thoracic Surgery. 2003;**75**:382-387

[35] Haciibrahimoglu G, Fazlioglu M, Olcmen A, Gurses A, Bedirhan MA. Surgical management of childhood bronchiectasis due to infectious disease. The Journal of Thoracic and Cardiovascular Surgery. 2004;**127**:1361-1365

[36] Otgun I, Karnak I, Tanyel FC, Senocak ME, Buyukpamukcu N. Surgical treatment of bronchiectasis in children. Journal of Pediatric Surgery. 2004;**39**:1532-1536

[37] Al-Kattan KM, Essa MA, Hajjar WM, Ashour MH, Saleh WN, Rafay MA. Surgical results for bronchiectasis based on hemodynamic (functional and morphologic) classification. The Journal of Thoracic and Cardiovascular Surgery. 2005;**130**:1385-1390

[38] Schneiter D, Meyer N, Lardinois D, Korom S, Kestenholz P, Weder W. Surgery for non-localized bronchiectasis. The British Journal of Surgery. 2005;**92**(7):836-839

[39] Aghajanzadeh M, Sarshad A, Amani H, Alavy A. Surgical management of bilateral bronchiectases: Results in 29 patients. Asian Cardiovascular & Thoracic Annals. 2006;**14**:219-222

[40] Yuncu G, Ceylan KC, Sevinc S, Ucvet A, Kaya SO, Kiter G, et al. Functional results of surgical treatment of bronchiectasis in a developing country. Archivos de Bronconeumología. 2006;**42**:183-188

[41] Eren S, Esme H, Avci A. Risk factors affecting outcome and morbidity in the surgical management of bronchiectasis. The Journal of Thoracic and Cardiovascular Surgery. 2007;**134**:392-398

[42] Guerra MS, Miranda JA, Leal F, Vouga L. Surgical treatment of bronchiectasis. Revista Portuguesa de Pneumologia. 2007;**13**(5):691-701

[43] Sirmali M, Karasu S, Turut H, Gezer S, Kaya S, Taştepe I, et al. Surgical management of bronchiectasis in childhood. European Journal of Cardio-Thoracic Surgery. 2007;**31**:120-123

[44] Stephen T, Thankachen R, Madhu AP, Neelakantan N, Shukla V, Korula RJ. Surgical results in bronchiectasis: Analysis of 149 patients. Asian Cardiovascular & Thoracic Annals. 2007;**15**:290-296

[45] Giovannetti R, Alifano M, Stefani A, Legras A, Grigoroiu M, Collet JY, et al. Surgical treatment of bronchiectasis: Early and long-term results. Interactive CardioVascular and Thoracic Surgery. 2008;**7**:609-612

[46] Bagheri R, Haghi SZ, Fattahi Masoum SH, Bahadorzadeh L. Surgical management of bronchiectasis: Analysis of 277 patients. The Thoracic and Cardiovascular Surgeon. 2010;**58**:291-294

[47] Gursoy S, Ozturk AA, Ucvet A, Erbaycu AE. Surgical management of bronchiectasis: The indications and outcomes. Surgery Today. 2010;**40**:26-30

[48] Zhang P, Jiang G, Ding J, Zhou X, Gao W. Surgical treatment of bronchiectasis: A retrospective analysis of 790 patients. The Annals of Thoracic Surgery. 2010;**90**:246-250

[49] Caylak H, Genc O, Kavakli K, Gurkok S, Gozubuyuk A, Yucel O, et al. Surgical management of bronchiectasis: A collective review of 339 patients with long-term follow-up. The Thoracic and Cardiovascular Surgeon. 2011;**59**:479-483

[50] Cobanoglu U, Yalcinkaya I, Er M, Isik AF, Sayir F, Mergan D. Surgery for bronchiectasis: The effect of morphological types to prognosis. Annals of Thoracic Medicine. 2011;**6**(1):25-32

[51] Gorur R, Turut H, Yiyit N, Candas F, Yildizhan A, Sen H, et al. The influence of specific factors on postoperative morbidity in young adults with bronchiectasis. Heart, Lung & Circulation. 2011;**20**:468-472

[52] Sehitogullari A, Bilici S, Sayir F, Cobanoglu U, Kahraman A. A long-term study assessing the factors influencing survival and morbidity in the surgical management of bronchiectasis. Journal of Cardiothoracic Surgery. 2011;**6**:161

[53] Hiramatsu M, Shiraishi Y, Nakajima Y, Miyaoka E, Katsuragi N, Kita H, et al. Risk factors that affect the surgical outcome in the management of focal bronchiectasis in a developed country. The Annals of Thoracic Surgery. 2012;**93**:245-250

[54] Al-Refaie RE, Amer S, El-Shabrawy M. Surgical treatment of bronchiectasis: A retrospective observational study of 138 patients. Journal of Thoracic Disease. 2013;**5**:228-233

[55] Zhou ZL, Zhao H, Li Y, Li JF, Jiang GC, Wang J. Completely thoracoscopic lobectomy for the surgical management of bronchiectasis. Chinese Medical Journal. 2013;**126**:875-878

[56] Andrade CF, Melo IA, Holand AR, Silva ÉF, Fischer GB, Felicetii JC. Surgical treatment of non-cystic fibrosis bronchiectasis in Brazilian children. Pediatric Surgery International. 2014;**30**:63-69

[57] Balci AE, Balci TA, Ozyurtan MO. Current surgical therapy for bronchiectasis: Surgical results and predictive factors in 86 patients. The Annals of Thoracic Surgery. 2014;**97**:211-217

[58] Jin YX, Zhang Y, Duan L, Yang Y, Jiang GN, Ding JA. Surgical treatment of bronchiectasis – A retrospective observational study of 260 patients. International Journal of Surgery. 2014;**12**:1050-1054

[59] Sahin A, Meteroglu F, Kelekci S, Karabel M, Eren C, Eren S, et al. Surgical outcome of bronchiectasis in children: Long term results of 60 cases. Klinische Pädiatrie. 2014;**226**:233-237

[60] Vallilo CC, Terra RM, de Albuquerque AL, Suesada MM, Mariani AW, Salge JM, et al. Lung resection improves the quality of life of patients with symptomatic bronchiectasis. The Annals of Thoracic Surgery. 2014;**98**:1034-1041

[61] Coutinho D, Fernandes P, Guerra M, Miranda J, Vouga L. Surgical treatment of bronchiectasis: A review of 20 years of experience. Revista Portuguesa de Pneumologia. 2016;**22**(2):82-85

[62] Baysungur V, Dogruyol T, Ocakcioglu I, Misirlioglu A, Evman S, Kanbur S, et al. The feasibility of thoracoscopic resection in bronchiectasis. Surgical Laparoscopy, Endoscopy & Percutaneous Techniques. 2017;**27**(3):194-196

[63] Dai J, Zhu X, Bian D, Fei K, Jiang G, Zhang P. Surgery for predominant lesion in nonlocalized bronchiectasis. The Thoracic and Cardiovascular Surgeon. 2017;**153**:979-985

[64] Hao X, Dazhong L, Lei Y, Jiaying Z, Linyou Z. Surgical treatment of

bronchiectasis: 5 years of experience at a single institution. Journal of Laparoendoscopic & Advanced Surgical Techniques. Part A. 2019;**29**(6):826-830

[65] Nega B, Ademe Y, Tizazu A. Bronchiectasis: Experience of surgical management at Tikur Anbessa specialized hospital, Addis Ababa, Ethiopia. Journal of Health Sciences. 2019;**29**(4):471-476. DOI: 10.4314/ejhs.v29i4.8

[66] Ocakcioglu I. Uniportal thoracoscopic treatment in bronchiectasis patients: Preliminary experience. Videosurgery and Other Miniinvasive Techniques. 2019;**14**(2):304-310

[67] Cantin L, Bankier AA, Eisenberg RL. Bronchiectasis. AJR. American Journal of Roentgenology. 2009;**193**(3):W158-W171

[68] van der Bruggen-Bogaarts BA, van der Bruggen HM, van Waes PF, Lammers JW. Screening for bronchiectasis. A comparative study between chest radiography and high-resolution CT. Chest. 1996;**109**(3):608-611

[69] Young K, Aspestrand F, Kolbenstvedt A. High resolution CT and bronchography in the assessment of bronchiectasis. Acta Radiologica. 1991;**32**:439-441

[70] Firth J. Respiratory medicine: Bronchiectasis. Clinical Medicine. 2019;**19**(1):64-67

[71] Ashour M. Hemodynamic alterations in bronchiectasis: A basis for a new subclassification of the disease. The Journal of Thoracic and Cardiovascular Surgery. 1996;**112**:328-334

[72] Dusica S, Nebojsa L, Miodrag M, Angelina B, Sveljko S, Radmilo J. Preoperative preparation of patients with infectious and restrictive respiratory diseases as comorbidities. Acta Chirurgica Iugoslavica. 2011;**58**(2):63-69

[73] Agasthian T. Surgery for bronchiectasis. Journal of Visceral Surgery. 2018;**4**:235

[74] O'Leary CJ, Wilson CB, Hansell DM, Cole PJ, Wilson R, Jones PW. Relationship between psychological well-being and lung health status in patients with bronchiectasis. Respiratory Medicine. 2002;**96**:686-692

[75] Olveira G, Olveira C, Gaspar I, Dorado A, Cruz I, Soriguer F, et al. Depression and anxiety symptoms in bronchiectasis: Associations with health-related quality of life. Quality of Life Research. 2013;**22**:597-665

[76] Artaraz A, Crichton ML, Finch S, Abo-Leyah H, Goeminne P, Aliberti S, et al. Development and initial validation of the bronchiectasis exacerbation and symptom tool (BEST). Respiratory Research. 2020;**21**(1):18

[77] McGovern EM, Trastek VF, Pairolero PC, Payne WS. Completion pneumonectomy: Indications, complications and results. The Annals of Thoracic Surgery. 1988;**46**:141-146

[78] Gregoire J, Deslauriers J, Guojin L, Rouleau J. Indications, risks, and results of completion pneumonectomy. The Journal of Thoracic and Cardiovascular Surgery. 1993;**105**:918-924

[79] McCallum GB, Binks MJ. The epidemiology of chronic suppurative lung disease and bronchiectasis in children and adolescents. Frontiers in Pediatrics. 2017;**5**:27

[80] Kumar A, Lodha R, Kumar P, Kabra SK. Non-cystic fibrosis bronchiectasis in children: Clinical profile, etiology and outcome. Indian Pediatrics. 2015;**52**(1):35-37